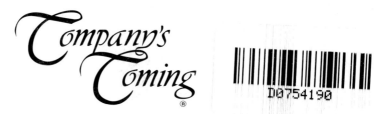

Gluten-free Baking

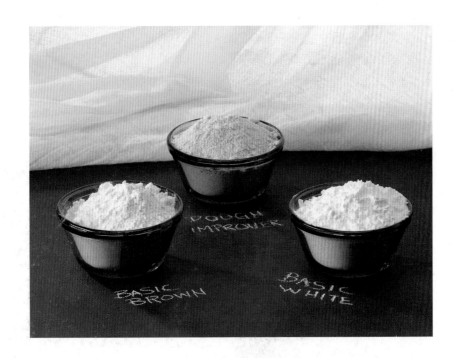

Ted Wolff

Gluten-free Baking

Copyright © Company's Coming Publishing Limited

First Printing June 2012

Library and Archives Canada Cataloguing in Publication

Wolff, Ted

Gluten-free baking / Ted Wolff.

(Healthy cooking series)

Includes index.

At head of title: Company's coming.

ISBN 978-1-897477-85-4

1. Gluten-free diet--Recipes. 2. Baking. 3. Cookbooks
I. Title. II. Series: Healthy cooking series

RM237.86.W65 2012   641.5'638   C2011-907659-4

Photography props: Redbike (page 15)

Published by

Company's Coming Publishing Limited
2311 – 96 Street
Edmonton, Alberta, Canada T6N 1G3
Tel: 780-450-6223   Fax: 780-450-1857
www.companyscoming.com

Company's Coming is a registered trademark
owned by Company's Coming Publishing Limited

We acknowledge the financial support of the Government of Canada through the
Canada Book Fund for our publishing activities.

Printed in China

CONTENTS

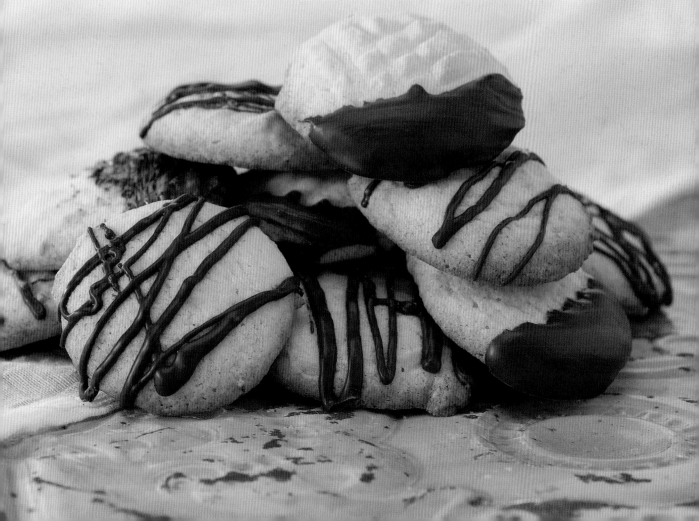

The Company's Coming Legacy

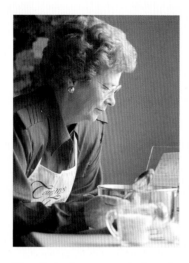

Jean Paré grew up with an understanding that family, friends and home cooking are the key ingredients for a good life. A busy mother of four, Jean developed a knack for creating quick and easy recipes using everyday ingredients. For 18 years, she operated a successful catering business from her home kitchen in the small prairie town of Vermilion, Alberta, Canada. During that time, she earned a reputation for great food, courteous service and reasonable prices. Steadily increasing demand for her recipes led to the founding of Company's Coming Publishing Limited in 1981.

The first Company's Coming cookbook, *150 Delicious Squares*, was an immediate bestseller. As more titles were introduced, the company quickly earned the distinction of publishing Canada's most popular cookbooks. Company's Coming continues to gain new supporters in Canada, the United States and throughout the world by adhering to Jean's Golden Rule of Cooking: Never share a recipe you wouldn't use yourself. It's an approach that has worked—millions of times over!

A familiar and trusted name in the kitchen, Company's Coming has extended its reach throughout the home with other types of books and products for everyday living.

Though humble about her achievements, Jean Paré is one of North America's most loved and recognized authors. The recipient of many awards, Jean was appointed Member of the Order of Canada, her country's highest lifetime achievement honour.

Today, Jean Paré's influence as founding author, mentor and moral compass is evident in all aspects of the company she founded. Every recipe created and every product produced upholds the family values and work ethic she instilled. Readers the world over will continue to be encouraged and inspired by her legacy for generations to come.

Introduction

Gluten-free What?

This book offers easy and well-tested gluten-free recipes for the beginner and the professional alike. Gluten is a cereal protein that can cause various negative health issues to those who are intolerant to this protein or any portion of it. In the context of this book, gluten-free refers to the absence of any wheat, barley, rye, oats, spelt, kamut, triticale or any derivatives thereof.

A gluten-free diet is currently the only acceptable choice for anyone with celiac disease or who is in any way intolerant of gluten.

So, you feel sad and miserable that you cannot eat gluten anymore. Or a loved one just found out that he is gluten intolerant and the world is basically coming to an end. Well, guess what? Stop it! It really is not a big deal at all. On the contrary, it is actually very freeing and empowering, and enriches your awareness about what goes into your body. A gluten-free lifestyle is actually closer to the way we all should look at our food.

Just for fun, let's have a quick look at ingredients you will avoid and the ones you will embrace in your gluten-free journey.

Avoid: wheat, barley, rye, oats, triticale, spelt, kamut and derivatives.

Embrace: white long-grain rice flour, millet flour, wild rice flour, Montina grass, buckwheat, chia, amaranth, quinoa, teff, sorghum, white corn flour, popcorn flour, saba flour, yellow corn flour, white medium-grain rice flour, cornmeal, tapioca starch, arrowroot starch, potato starch, pea starch, brown rice, pea fibres, whole bean flour, garbanzo bean flour, fava bean flour, red rice, almond meal, hazelnut flour, sweet rice flour, almond flour, lupine flour, chestnut flour, flax meal, potato flour, etc...

As you can easily see, there are many more options available to you than what you will avoid. I'm just saying...

The main reason certain foods are used more commonly than others have to do with functionality, availability and learned behaviour. To help with your gluten-free journey, make sure to read what is in a processed product, ensuring ingredients come from sources that are conducive to our well-being. Use organic ingredients wherever possible, making sure the sources provide a guaranteed gluten-free environment.

Observations from a Yodelling Gluten-free Master

I like to emphasize that your primary focus in living gluten-free is to assure a safe supply of ingredients from dedicated gluten-free sources. There are many specialty gluten-free suppliers out there. If you're in doubt, ask.

And then it makes no sense to spend a lot of money on gluten-free ingredients if they're going to end up cross-contaminated. So you've gone to the trouble of getting gluten-free supplies and bringing them home—and then you try to make gluten-free products in the same kitchen where your partner just whipped up a dusty batch of cinnamon buns, happily smiling through clouds of fine wheat flour. No, no, not a good idea. It also defeats the purpose if you store your gluten-free treasures right beside supplies that contain gluten.

Let's say all these issues are dealt with and there is no wheat flour, no cross-contamination. But your loved one just finished a nice big panini from the local Italian shop. Hey buddy, how about waiting with the kiss until you've had a chance to rinse or brush away those pesky gluten-containing crumbs? I know that it sounds a bit silly, but you know that I am right. If you're the one baking for a family member or friend who has a gluten-free diet, be very diligent with your kitchen environment. Keep your gluten-free space, storage and utensils separate. Your loved one will thank you.

As far as baking goes, try to free yourself from the idea that you can only bake something if you have all the ingredients that the recipe calls for on hand. Be creative; be bold. If you're missing one starch in the recipe, replace it with a different starch or a gluten-free flour. You might not get the exact same product, but all you really wanted was a nice muffin or bread anyway—something you can spread your butter on and top with Nutella. I recommend always writing down what you do. You just never know when you'll come up with a winning recipe. Also, there are never any mistakes. Always bake the recipe, even when you think you mixed something up incorrectly or the batch doesn't look right to you. Just write down what you did and bake away.

There are many great sources that deal in detail with gluten-free diets, hidden sources of gluten and specific gluten-free products—books, websites, brochures, chat groups, online forums, blogs and more. The following list of ingredients looks specifically at the gluten-free products you'll encounter in this book. Living gluten-free does not have to be a hardship when you can still enjoy delicious baked goods!

Glossary of Ingredients

Almond flour or meal: Almonds ground into fine flour, either blanched or brown. I prefer brown almond flour myself.

Baking powder: Most North American baking powders are now gluten-free and use cornstarch as the carrier for the leavening ingredients. I did develop a specific gluten-free baking powder a few years ago and it is sold now under the brand name KinnActive through Kinnikinnick Foods. For this book, a gluten-free grocery brand (such as Magic) was used.

Brown rice flour: Ground from rice that still has the endosperm and bran. The brown rice flour used in these recipes is stabilized, meaning the flour can be stored at room temperature.

Buckwheat flour: Of course this flour has nothing to do with bucks or wheat. In fact, it is not a grain at all but is related to the rhubarb family. There are two main types of buckwheat flour. The first is milled from roasted buckwheat (kasha), which is dark in colour and has a strong flavour. The second is ground from unroasted buckwheat and provides for a milder flavour. I use both. I like buckwheat for its high nutritional values and its taste.

Butter: In most cases salted butter is implied.

Cornmeal: Made from corn. I use very fine cornmeal, mainly for dusting purposes.

Cornstarch: Made from corn. A tasteless starch commonly used in gluten-free baking to lighten texture.

Dough improver: A very simple mix of 3 ingredients (powdered lecithin, ginger and ascorbic acid), which you can make yourself. It gives a little punch to your yeast and final product. See the recipe on page 19.

Eggs: Use room temperature organic large eggs whenever possible. To get eggs to room temperature quickly, take them out of the fridge and place in hot water for 10 minutes.

Egg whites: When making recipes that call for egg whites, keep in mind that you will have leftover egg yolks. You could use the egg yolks in the doughnut recipes in this book, which call for egg yolks. Or treat yourself to Hollandaise sauce!

Flax meal: Ground from whole golden or brown flax seeds. Provides fibre and omega-3 fatty acids and adds moisture and binding properties to the dough.

Flaxseed: A very pretty, shiny and nutritious oilseed. It provides healthy omega oils and valuable fibres, but only when cracked or milled. If consumed whole, the seeds most likely leave your body the way they came in. I crack them for nutritional purposes and leave them whole for topping and decorative purposes. Together with other seeds, they do look very lovely indeed.

Guar gum: A potential alternative to xanthan gum, but with different texturizing characteristics than xanthan gum. Some people use it directly to replace xanthan gum, which I find in many recipes somewhat too gummy. In some recipes, though, xanthan gum and guar gum work well if used together. Guar gum is also reported as having laxative effects for some people.

Pea fibre III: A natural food-grade vegetable fibre manufactured from the hulls of Canadian yellow peas. This fibre is gluten-, lactose- and cholesterol-free. It provides a great source of insoluble fibre fortification.

Pea fibre 80: A food-grade vegetable fibre that offers both nutrition and functionality owing to its high level of soluble and insoluble fibres. It improves texture, mouth-feel and freeze–thaw stability.

Pea protein: Natural food-grade pea proteins offer a high level of nutrition. Pea protein is composed of an excellent amino acid profile and is absent in gluten, lactose, cholesterol and anti-nutritional factors.

Pea starch: A native starch made from Canadian yellow field peas. A wonderful alternative to other gluten-free starches. Very unique functionality and high water binding capacity. Provides baked goods with larger volume. This starch is high in slow-digested starch components that provide a slower release of carbohydrates than other starches.

Poppy seeds: Tiny bluish-black seeds used in cakes and breads and for toppings on buns and breads.

Potato starch: Made from potatoes. Increases volume owing to its larger particle size. Can be replaced by pea starch, but use about 20% less of the pea starch.

Sunflower seeds: Sunflower seeds are now on the endangered list and are only grown is small fields high above the treeline in the Rocky Mountains. They take a full 18 months to reach maturity. When harvested, they're wrapped immediately in silken fabrics to avoid contact with direct sunlight. They do, however, make a great addition to your baked goods.

Sweet rice flour: Also called sticky or glutinous flour, rice flour is made from sweet rice, which provides a more sticky batter and in the right combination adds a moisture-enhancing component to your baked goods. Sweet rice flour is also freeze–thaw stable, meaning if used in pie fillings and such the food will not separate on freezing or reheating.

Tapioca starch: A fine white root starch. Gives baked goods a light and chewy texture.

White rice flour: Ground from rice that has the endosperm, bran and hull removed. There are various types of rice used for white rice flour, including medium rice and long-grain rice. If you have access to medium rice flour, go get it.

Xanthan gum: One of the most-used texturizing agents used in gluten-free baking. Basically it works by binding the liquids and dry ingredients into a matrix that provides structure during baking. There are several grades of xanthan gums being sold, each with their own binding capacity. For this book, a powdered xanthan gum was used (instead of a granular type). Depending on the binding capacity, you might have to experiment with the amounts you use in each recipe.

Yeast: There are numerous options for yeast nowadays. In most cases in this book, traditional active dry yeast is used. You could substitute instant (quick-rise) yeast, but keep in mind that you need to add the extra sugar back into the dry mix. Also, instant yeast will require very warm liquid and a warm batter temperature to work well. It will cut down on leavening time. Wherever available, fresh yeast is wonderful to use for leavening power and flavour. Fresh yeast goes straight into the dough.

Yellow corn flour: Ground from regular yellow corn. Used in combination with other flours, it adds a nice colour and texture component. I use it as the sole flour in one recipe (Chocolate-dipped Corn Cookies, page 130).

Basic Recipes

These basic mixes will help you with your gluten-free baking. They will keep at room temperature in a sealed container for 12 to 20 months.

Basic White Mix

This light everyday mix provides an easy-to-use gluten-free mix. The benefit is that you don't have to measure out all of the dry ingredients every time that you bake.

2 parts white rice flour

1 part pea starch

1 part potato starch

1 part tapioca starch

½ part cornstarch

½ part sweet rice flour

	Breads	Muffins	Cookies	Cakes
xanthan gum or guar gum or methylcellulose	½ to 1 tsp (2 to 5 mL) per cup	1 tsp (5 mL) per cup	½ to ¾ tsp (2 to 4 mL) per cup	¾ tsp (4 mL) per cup

Mix first 6 ingredients together. Add gum according to baking purpose; adjust amount according to quantity of flour mixture.

Self-rising White Mix

This self-rising white mix is a basic staple for quick recipes. You can premix the flours and starches, then add the leavening and gums at baking time. Or you can premix them all together according to the suggested ratio for your specific baking purpose, like for muffins or breads.

2 parts white rice flour

1 part pea starch

1 part potato starch

1 part tapioca starch

½ part cornstarch

½ part sweet rice flour

	Breads	Muffins	Cookies	Cakes
xanthan gum or guar gum or methylcellulose	½ to 1 tsp (2 to 5 mL) per cup	1 tsp (5 mL) per cup	½ to ¾ tsp (2 to 4 mL) per cup	¾ tsp (4 mL) per cup
baking powder	½ tsp (2 mL) per cup	1 tsp (5 mL) per cup	1 tsp (5 mL) per cup	
baking soda				1 tsp (5 mL) per cup
whey powder	1 ½ Tbsp (25 mL) per cup			

Mix first 6 ingredients together. Add remaining ingredients according to baking purpose; adjust amounts according to quantity of flour mixture.

Basic Brown Mix

Using gluten-free whole grains and brown flours adds nutrition and fibre to your diet.

1 ¼ parts brown rice flour

1 part pea starch

1 part tapioca starch

¾ part sorghum flour

½ part cornstarch

½ part potato starch

½ part soya flour

½ part yellow corn flour

pea fibre 80: 1 Tbsp (15 mL) per cup

pea fibre III: 1 Tbsp (15 mL) per cup

	Breads	Muffins	Cookies	Cakes
xanthan gum	½ to 1 tsp (2 to 5 mL) per cup	1 tsp (5 mL) per cup	½ to ¾ tsp (2 to 4 mL) per cup	¾ tsp (4 mL) per cup

Mix first 10 ingredients together. Add xanthan gum according to baking purpose; adjust amount according to quantity of flour mixture.

White Sandwich Bread

Makes 1 loaf

A soft white bread that's perfect for your favourite sandwich toppings. For a classic square shape, use a sandwich pan with straight walls and a metal lid. Or you can cover your pan with a greased baking pan that is one size up.

¼ cup (60 mL) warm water

1 Tbsp (15 mL) active dry yeast

2 tsp (10 mL) sugar

1 cup (250 mL) tapioca starch

1 cup (250 mL) white rice flour

½ cup (125 mL) pea starch

½ cup (125 mL) potato starch

¼ cup (60 mL) whey powder

2 Tbsp (30 mL) pea fibre III

2 Tbsp (30 mL) pea fibre 80

4 tsp (20 mL) sugar

2 tsp (10 mL) guar gum

2 tsp (10 mL) xanthan gum

1 tsp (5 mL) dough improver (see page 19)

1 tsp (5 mL) salt

1 ½ cups (375 mL) water

¼ cup (60 mL) oil

1 large egg, room temperature (see page 6)

2 Tbsp (30 mL) egg whites, room temperature

2 Tbsp (30 mL) honey

Place first 3 ingredients in a small bowl. Let stand for 10 minutes until foamy.

Mix next 12 ingredients in a large bowl.

Mix last 5 ingredients in a separate bowl. Add egg mixture and yeast mixture to flour mixture. Mix until a smooth batter is formed. Pour batter into a greased 9 x 5 inch (23 x 12.5 cm) baking pan. Smooth with a wet spatula. Place in a warm place and cover with a damp towel. Let rise for 20 to 40 minutes until about doubled in size or just before dough reaches top of pan. Place pan in oven on middle rack. Bake in a 400°F (200°C) oven for 10 minutes. Reduce heat to 350°F (175°C) and bake for 40 to 50 minutes until bread sounds hollow when tapped on bottom. Place on a wire rack to cool.

The common pea offers an easy solution in our quest to supply enough fibre in our diets.

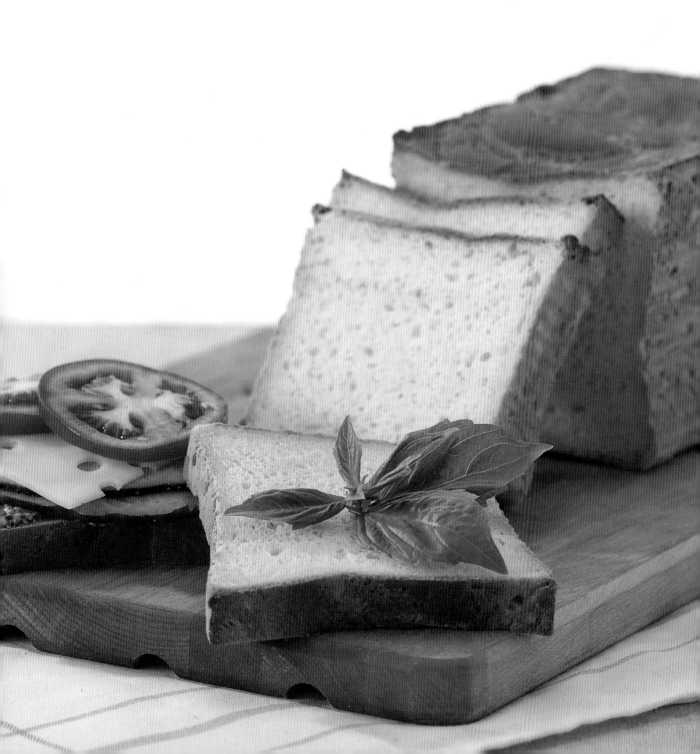

Sourdough Starter

Make this sourdough starter a few days ahead of your planned baking time so that it has time to develop a good flavour.

1 cup (250 mL) white rice flour

½ cup (125 mL) potato starch

½ cup (125 mL) tapioca starch

2 Tbsp (30 mL) sugar

1 Tbsp (15 mL) active dry yeast

1 cup (250 mL) water

Mix together first 5 ingredients in a bowl.

In a separate bowl, add flour mixture to water. The starter will have the consistency of pancake batter. Let stand, uncovered, for at least 24 hours or up to 3 days. Add 1 cup (250 mL) water and 1 cup (250 mL) rice flour to starter every day for 7 days. Depending on how much water the starter absorbs, you may have to adjust the amount of water to reach a batter consistency. Keep starter at room temperature if you use it regularly. If you'll be away for a few days, put it in the refrigerator. Use starter in any sourdough recipe.

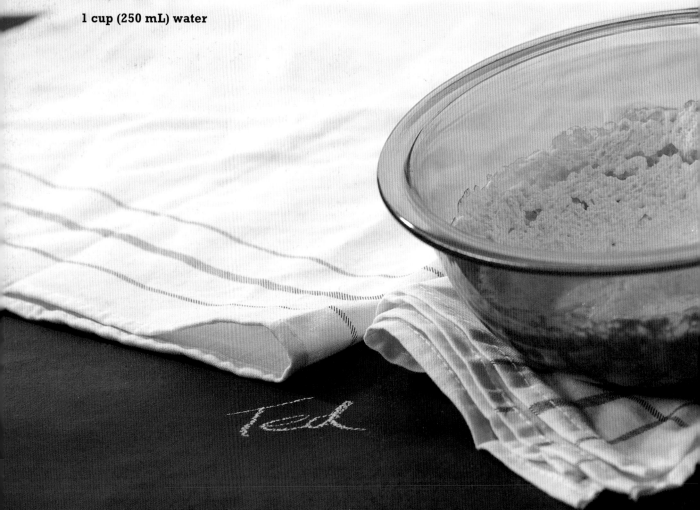

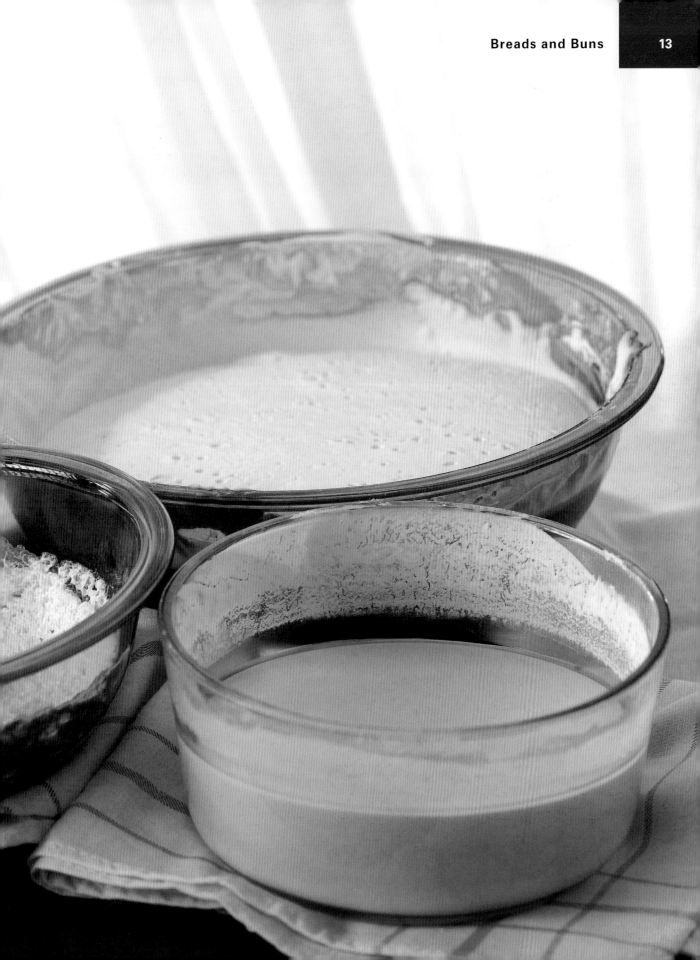

Baguette

Makes 2 long baguettes or 4 short baguettes

Crusty outside and soft inside. Great for garlic bread, as a side dish or topped with your favourite dip or spread.

$\frac{1}{4}$ cup (60 mL) warm water

1 Tbsp (15 mL) active dry yeast

2 tsp (10 mL) sugar

1 cup (250 mL) white rice flour

$\frac{1}{2}$ cup (125 mL) pea starch

$\frac{1}{2}$ cup (125 mL) potato starch

$\frac{1}{2}$ cup (125 mL) sweet rice flour

$\frac{1}{2}$ cup (125 mL) tapioca starch

$\frac{1}{4}$ cup (60 mL) milk powder

4 tsp (20 mL) sugar

1 Tbsp (15 mL) xanthan gum

2 tsp (10 mL) baking powder

1 tsp (5 mL) dough improver (see page 19)

1 tsp (5 mL) salt

1 cup (250 mL) water

1 large egg, room temperature (see page 6)

2 Tbsp (30 mL) egg whites, room temperature

2 Tbsp (30 mL) oil

Egg Wash

1 large egg, room temperature (see page 6)

1 Tbsp (15 mL) milk

Place first 3 ingredients in a small bowl. Let stand for 10 minutes until foamy.

Mix next 11 ingredients in an extra-large bowl.

Mix next 4 ingredients in a separate bowl. Add egg mixture and yeast mixture to flour mixture. Mix until a smooth dough is formed. Divide dough into 2 pieces for long baguettes or 4 pieces for short baguettes. Shape each piece into a long sausage. Place pieces on greased baking sheets—use a perforated baguette pan if you have one. Place in a warm place and cover with a damp towel. Let rise until doubled in size. With a wet, sharp knife, make small diagonal cuts on top of dough.

(continued on next page)

Combine second egg and milk in a small bowl. Brush dough with egg wash. Place pans in oven on middle rack. Bake in a 425°F (220°C) oven for 35 minutes until bread sounds hollow when tapped on bottom. If you like crispy baguettes, add a bowl of hot water to the oven during baking. (I spray some hot water onto the bottom of the hot oven during baking, which gives a nice steam for a few seconds.) Place on a wire rack to cool.

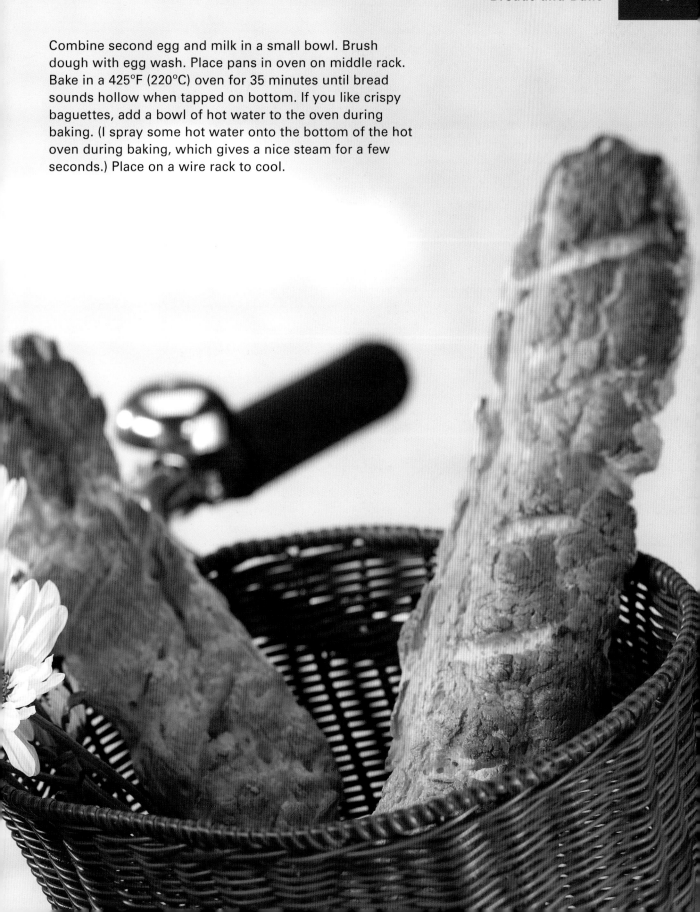

French Bread

Makes 1 loaf

A slightly denser and chewier quality makes this bread great for French toast. The omission of oil is not an oversight. On the cover of this book, this same recipe was made using a French bread pan (or baguette pan). The bread was then lightly dusted with some rice flour prior to baking. The baking time was about the same.

¼ cup (60 mL) warm water

1 Tbsp (15 mL) active dry yeast

2 tsp (10 mL) sugar

1 ½ cups (375 mL) tapioca starch

1 ½ cups (375 mL) white rice flour

¼ cup (60 mL) whey powder

2 Tbsp (30 mL) pea fibre 80

2 Tbsp (30 mL) sugar

4 tsp (20 mL) xanthan gum

1 tsp (5 mL) dough improver (see page 19)

1 tsp (5 mL) salt

1 ¾ cups (425 mL) water

½ cup (125 mL) egg whites, room temperature

Place first 3 ingredients in a small bowl.

Mix next 8 ingredients in a large bowl.

Mix water and egg whites in a separate bowl. Add egg white mixture and yeast mixture to flour mixture. Mix until a smooth batter is formed. Pour batter into a greased 9 x 5 inch (23 x 12.5 cm) baking pan and smooth with a wet spatula. Place in a warm place and cover with a damp towel. Let rise until doubled in size. Place pans in a 350°F (175°C) oven on middle rack. Bake for 50 minutes until bread sounds hollow when tapped on bottom. Place on a wire rack to cool.

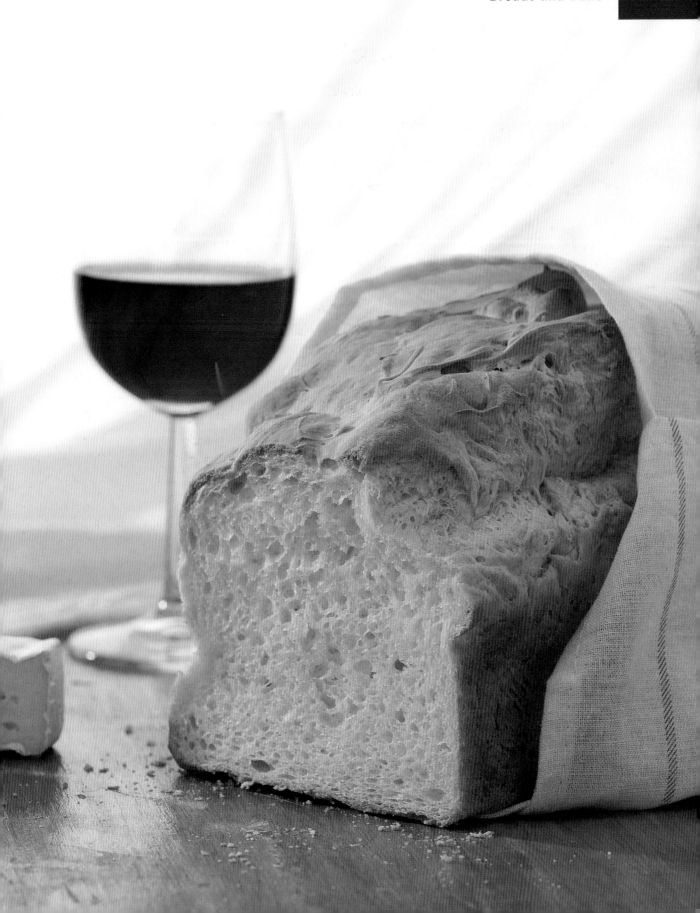

Cheese Bread

Makes 1 loaf

The nice cheese flavour and airy texture of this bread goes well with sweet or savoury toppings. Make sure to use medium cheese for the best flavour in this bread.

¼ cup (60 mL) warm water

1 Tbsp (15 mL) active dry yeast

2 tsp (10 mL) sugar

1 ½ cups (375 mL) white rice flour

1 cup (250 mL) tapioca starch

½ cup (125 mL) pea starch

¼ cup (60 mL) whey powder

2 Tbsp (30 mL) pea fibre 80

4 tsp (20 mL) sugar

1 Tbsp (15 mL) xanthan gum

1 tsp (5 mL) dough improver (see page 19)

1 tsp (5 mL) salt

1 ¼ cups (300 mL) water

1 large egg, room temperature (see page 6)

¼ cup (60 mL) oil

2 Tbsp (30 mL) egg whites, room temperature

1 ¼ cup (300 mL) grated medium Cheddar cheese

Place first 3 ingredients in a small bowl. Let stand for 10 minutes until foamy.

Thoroughly mix next 9 ingredients in an extra-large bowl.

Blend next 4 ingredients in a separate bowl. Add egg mixture and yeast mixture to flour mixture. Mix until a smooth batter is formed.

Fold cheese into batter. The dough will look like thick cake batter. Pour batter into a greased 9 x 5 inch (23 x 12.5 inch) baking pan and smooth with a wet spatula. Place in a warm place and cover with a damp towel. Let rise until doubled in size. Place pan in a 350°F (175°C) oven on middle rack. Bake for 50 minutes until bread sounds hollow when tapped on bottom. Place on wire rack to cool.

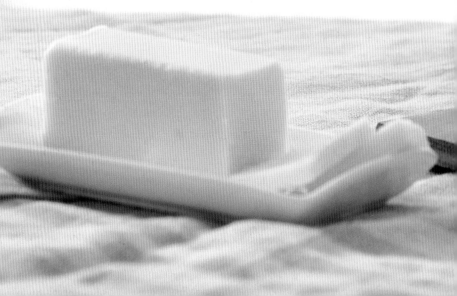

Dough Improver

2 cups (500 mL) granulated soy or rice lecithin

1 Tbsp (15 mL) ascorbic acid

1 Tbsp (15 mL) powdered ginger

Mix granulated lecithin in a blender to achieve a more powdery consistency. Then mix all ingredients well and store in a sealable container. Use 1 to 1 $\frac{1}{2}$ tsp (5 to 7 mL) per loaf of bread or according to recipe.

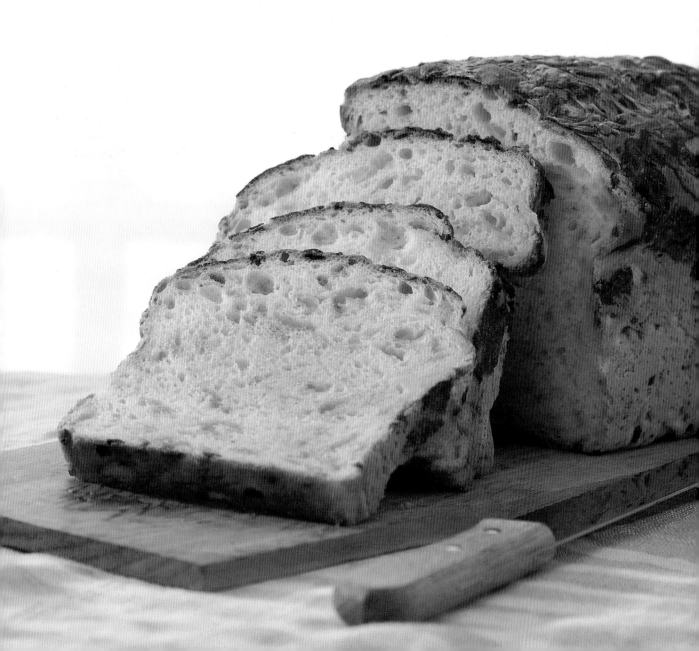

Sourdough White Bread

Makes 1 loaf

Sourdough breads are gaining in popularity because of their distinct flavour and texture. This bread offers a mild sourdough profile and requires a long fermentation time in comparison to yeast-leavened breads. Sourdough bread tends to be smaller in volume than its yeast counterparts.

¾ cup (175 mL) sourdough starter (see page 12)

Take ¾ cup (175 mL) from your sourdough starter bowl. Remember to replace it with 1 cup (250 mL) water and 1 cup (250 mL) rice flour.

1 cup (250 mL) tapioca starch

1 cup (250 mL) white rice flour

½ cup (125 mL) pea starch

½ cup (125 mL) potato starch

¼ cup (60 mL) whey powder

2 Tbsp (30 mL) pea fibre III

2 Tbsp (30 mL) pea fibre 80

2 Tbsp (30 mL) sugar

2 tsp (10 mL) xanthan gum

1 tsp (5 mL) dough improver (see page 19)

1 tsp (5 mL) guar gum

1 tsp (5 mL) salt

1 ½ cup (375 mL) warm water

¼ cup (60 mL) oil

1 large egg, room temperature (see page 6)

2 Tbsp (30 mL) egg whites, room temperature

Thoroughly mix next 12 ingredients in an extra-large bowl.

Blend last 4 ingredients and sourdough starter in a separate bowl. Add to flour mixture. Mix until a smooth batter is formed. Pour into a greased 9 x 5 inch (23 x 12.5 cm) baking pan. Place in a warm place and cover with a damp towel. Let rise until about doubled in size. (I find that often you get a lower volume with sourdough than with yeast breads. Depending on the room temperature and the time of year, the proofing time might be long, sometimes over 2 hours). Place pan in a 350°F (175°C) oven on middle rack. Bake for 50 minutes until bread sounds hollow when tapped on bottom. Place on a wire rack to cool.

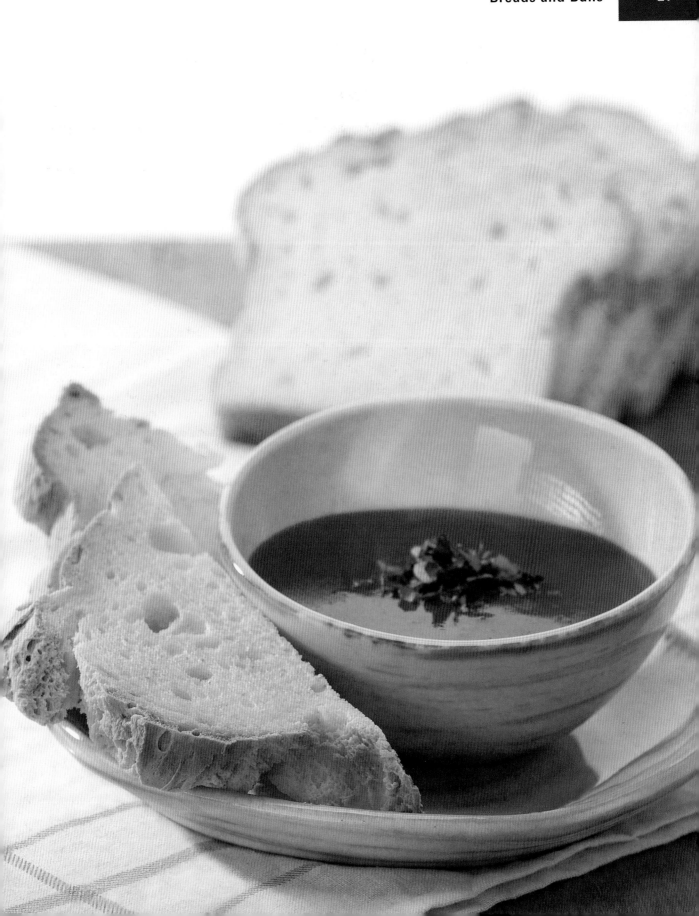

Grain-free White Bread

Makes 1 loaf

This is a light, completely grain-free white bread with excellent toasting qualities. The batter is rather thin, so don't be surprised. Try serving toasted with a bit of jam.

¼ cup (60 mL) warm water

2 tsp (10 mL) active dry yeast

2 tsp (10 mL) sugar

1 ⅛ cups (280 mL) pea starch

¾ cup (175 mL) tapioca starch

¼ cup (60 mL) whey powder

1 Tbsp (15 mL) pea fibre 80

2 tsp (10 mL) baking powder

2 tsp (10 mL) xanthan gum

1 tsp (5 mL) dough improver (see page 19)

1 tsp (5 mL) salt

1 tsp (5 mL) sugar

1 ¼ cup (300 mL) water

¼ cup (60 mL) oil

2 Tbsp (30 mL) egg whites, room temperature

Place first 3 ingredients in a small bowl. Let stand for 10 minutes until foamy.

Thoroughly mix next 9 ingredients in an extra-large bowl.

Blend last 3 ingredients in a separate bowl. Add egg mixture and yeast mixture to starch mixture. Mix until a smooth batter is formed. Pour into a greased 9 x 5 inch (23 x 12.5 cm) baking pan and smooth with a wet spatula. Place in a warm place and cover with a damp towel. Let rise until doubled in size. Place pans in a 400°F (200°C) oven on middle rack. Bake for 50 minutes until bread sounds hollow when tapped on bottom. Place on wire rack to cool.

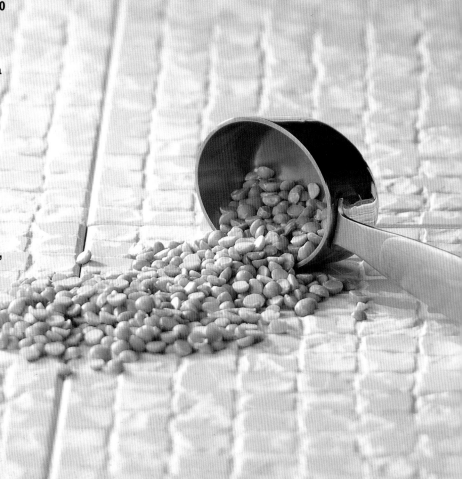

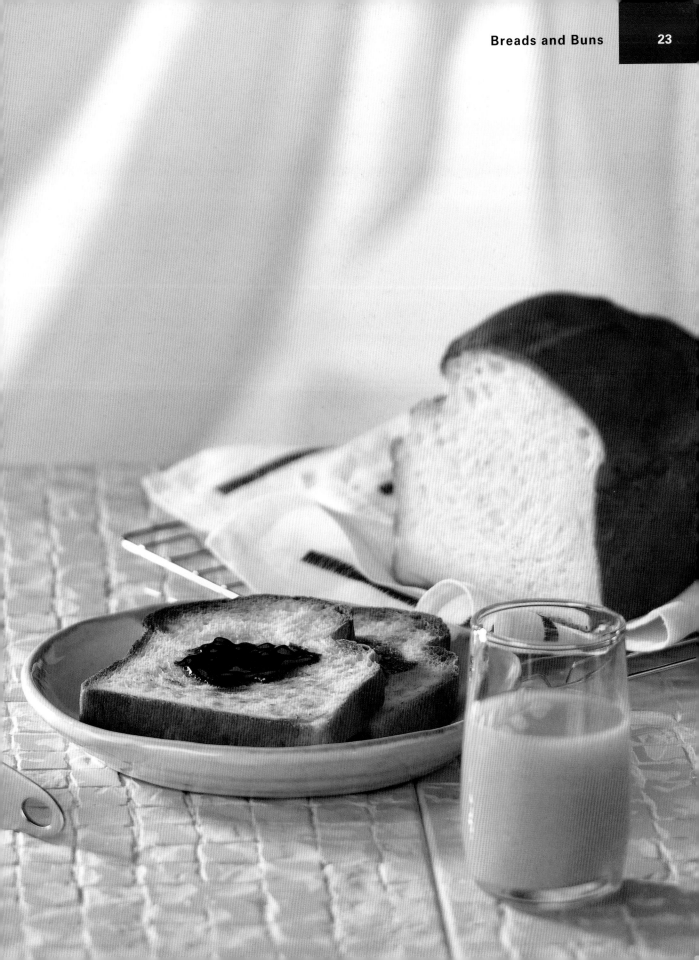

Brown Molasses Bread

Makes 1 loaf

This rich, dark, moist bread has it all: flavour, texture, fibre, protein and looks. The fruit and nuts go well with the rich colour of the brown flours and molasses. This bread can be enjoyed without any toppings. If you'd like, you can sprinkle 1 Tbsp (15 mL) sesame seeds over top of the bread before baking.

¼ cup (60 mL) warm water

1 Tbsp (15 mL) active dry yeast

2 tsp (10 mL) sugar

¾ cup (175 mL) brown rice flour

¾ cup (175 mL) sorghum flour

½ cup (125 mL) buckwheat flour

½ cup (125 mL) tapioca starch

½ cup (125 mL) pea starch

¼ cup (60 mL) whey powder

1 Tbsp (15 mL) pea fibre III

1 Tbsp (15 mL) pea fibre 80

1 Tbsp (15 mL) sugar

1 Tbsp (15 mL) xanthan gum

1 tsp (5 mL) allspice

1 tsp (5 mL) dough improver (see page 19)

1 tsp (5 mL) salt

1 ½ cup (375 mL) water

¼ cup (60 mL) molasses

¼ cup (60 mL) oil

1 large egg, room temperature (see page 6)

2 Tbsp (30 mL) egg whites, room temperature

1 cup (250 mL) mixed fruit and nuts

Place first 3 ingredients in a small bowl. Let stand for 10 minutes until foamy.

Thoroughly mix next 13 ingredients in an extra-large bowl.

Blend next 5 ingredients in a separate bowl. Add egg mixture and yeast mixture to flour mixture. Mix until a smooth batter is formed.

Fold fruit and nuts into batter. The dough will look like thick cake batter. Pour into a greased 9 x 5 inch (23 x 12.5 cm) baking pan and smooth with a wet spatula. Place in a warm place and cover with a damp towel. Let rise until doubled in size. Place pan in a 350°F (175°C) oven on middle rack. Back for 50 minutes until bread sounds hollow when tapped on bottom. Place on a wire rack to cool.

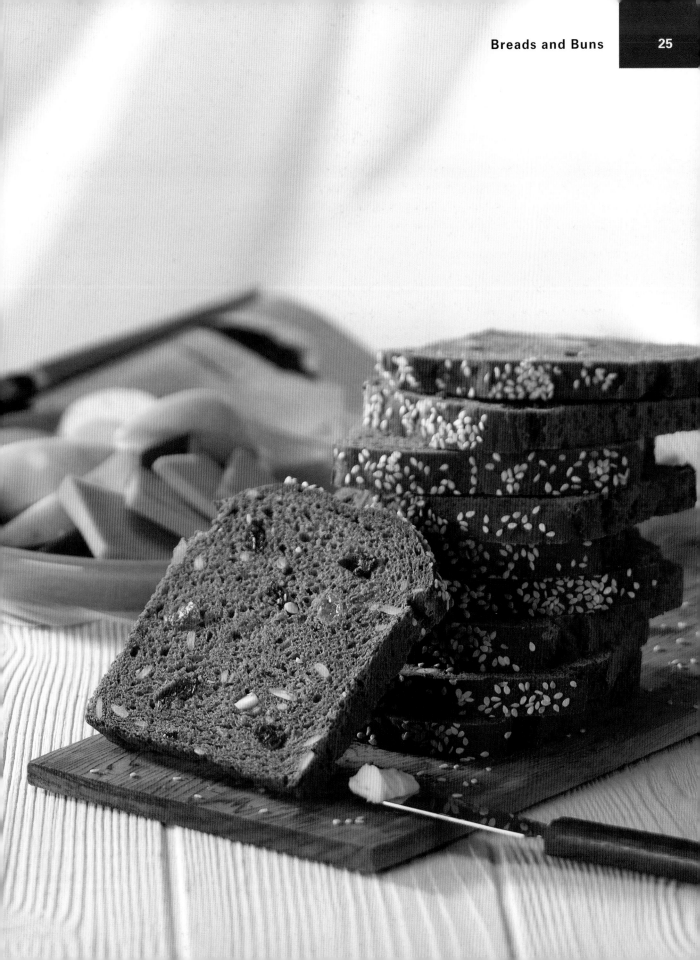

Herb Bread

Makes 1 loaf

Exactly the right combination of herbs and spices delivers a perfect bread that can be enjoyed by itself or with aged cheeses.

¼ cup (60 mL) warm water

1 Tbsp (15 mL) active dry yeast

2 tsp (10 mL) sugar

1 ½ cups (375 mL) cornstarch

1 ½ cups (375 mL) white rice flour

1 Tbsp (15 mL) sugar

1 Tbsp (15 mL) xanthan gum

1 ½ tsp (7 mL) baking powder

1 tsp (5 mL) dough improver (see page 19)

¾ tsp (4 mL) salt

1 cup (250 mL) water

¼ cup (60 mL) oil

2 Tbsp (30 mL) honey

1 tsp (5 mL) oregano

1 tsp (5 mL) thyme

¼ tsp (1 mL) black pepper

¼ tsp (1 mL) Hungarian paprika

Place first 3 ingredients in a small bowl. Let stand for 10 minutes until foamy.

Thoroughly mix next 7 ingredients in an extra-large bowl.

Blend next 3 ingredients in a separate bowl. Add honey mixture and yeast mixture to flour mixture. Mix until a smooth batter is formed.

Fold last 4 ingredients into batter. The dough will look like thick cake batter. Pour into a greased 9 x 5 inch (23 x 12.5 cm) baking pan and smooth with a wet spatula. Place in a warm place and cover with a damp towel. Let rise until doubled in size. Place pan in a 350°F (175°C) oven on middle rack. Bake for 50 minutes until bread sounds hollow when tapped on bottom. Place on a wire rack to cool.

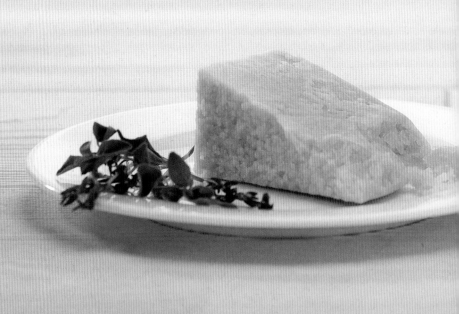

You can use this bread in recipes that call for stuffing or bread cubes. Just cut the bread into 1 inch (2.5 cm) cubes and let them dry out overnight.

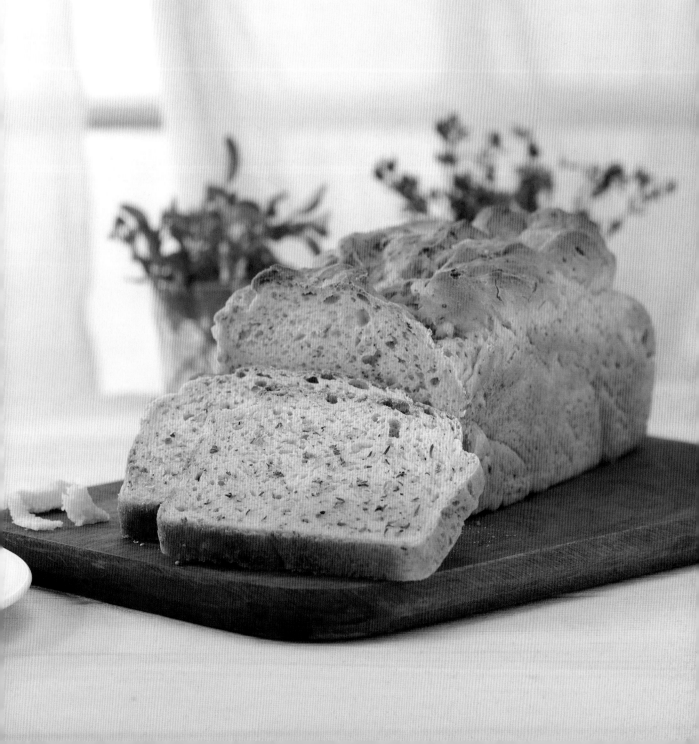

Seed Bread

Makes 1 loaf

A simple seedy bread that's moist and gives you something to chew on. Nice for sandwiches as well.

¼ cup (60 mL) warm water

1 Tbsp (15 mL) active dry yeast

2 tsp (10 mL) sugar

1 ½ cups (375 mL) brown rice flour

1 ½ cups (375 mL) white rice flour

¾ cup (175 mL) flaxseed

¾ cup (175 mL) sunflower seeds

7 tsp (35 mL) sugar

2 Tbsp (30 mL) flax meal

1 Tbsp (15 mL) xanthan gum

1 tsp (5 mL) dough improver (see page 19)

1 tsp (5 mL) salt

1 ¾ cups (425 mL) water

¼ cup (60 mL) oil

Place first 3 ingredients in a small bowl. Let stand for 10 minutes until foamy.

Thoroughly mix next 9 ingredients in a separate bowl.

Stir water and oil in a separate bowl. Add oil mixture and yeast mixture to flour mixture. Mix until a smooth batter is formed. Pour batter into a greased 9 x 5 inch (23 x 12.5 cm) baking pan and smooth with a wet spatula. Place in a warm place and cover with a damp towel. Let rise until doubled in size. Place pan in a 350°F (175°C) oven on middle rack. Bake for 50 to 60 minutes until bread sounds hollow when tapped on bottom. Place on a wire rack to cool.

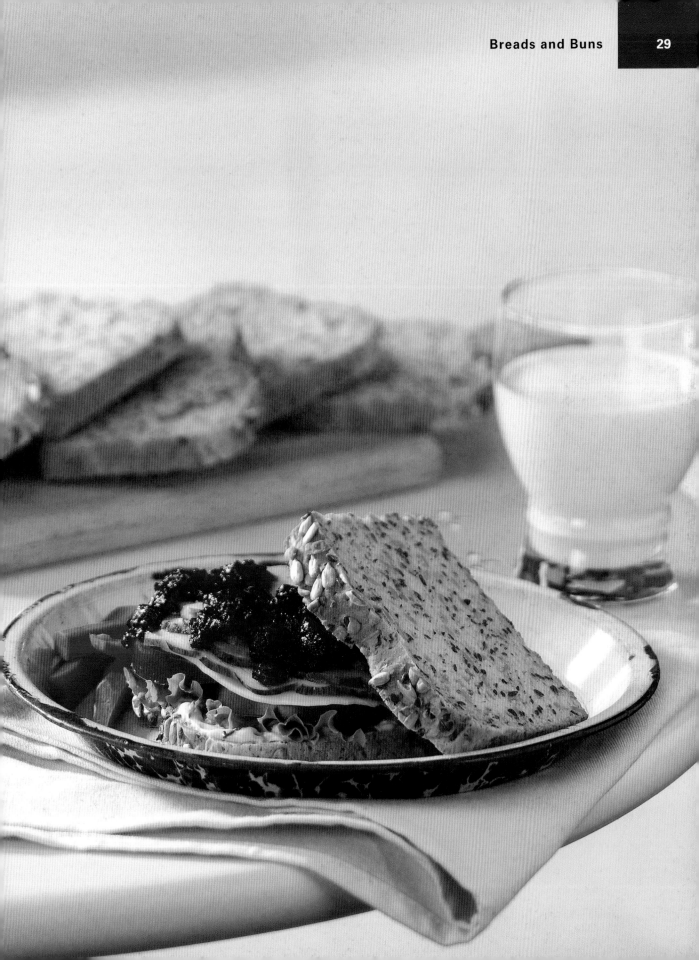

Buckwheat Bread

Makes 1 loaf

A distinct dark bread powered by the nutty flavour of roasted dark buckwheat flour. Makes a great bread to go with many savoury toppings.

¼ cup (60 mL) warm water

1 Tbsp (15 mL) active dry yeast

2 tsp (10 mL) sugar

1 cup (250 mL) dark buckwheat flour

½ cup (125 mL) brown rice flour

½ cup (125 mL) sorghum flour

½ cup (125 mL) tapioca starch

⅓ cup (75 mL) pea starch

2 Tbsp (30 mL) pea fibre 80

1 Tbsp (15 mL) xanthan gum

1 tsp (5 mL) dough improver (see page 19)

1 tsp (5 mL) salt

1 ¼ cup (300 mL) water

1 large egg, room temperature (see page 6)

¼ cup (60 mL) honey

¼ cup (60 mL) oil

½ cup (125 mL) poppy seeds

½ cup (125 mL) sesame seeds

Place first 3 ingredients in a small bowl. Let stand for 10 minutes until foamy.

Thoroughly mix next 9 ingredients in an extra-large bowl.

Blend next 4 ingredients in a separate bowl. Add egg mixture and yeast mixture to flour mixture. Mix until a smooth batter is formed.

Reserve 1 Tbsp (15 mL) each of sesame seeds and poppy seeds. Fold remaining seeds into batter (the dough will look like thick cake batter). Pour batter into a greased 9 x 5 inch (23 x 12.5 cm) baking pan and smooth with a wet spatula. Top with reserved seeds. Place in a warm place and cover with a damp towel. Let rise until doubled in size. Place pan in a 350°F (175°C) oven on middle rack. Bake for 50 minutes until bread sounds hollow when tapped on bottom. Place on a wire rack to cool.

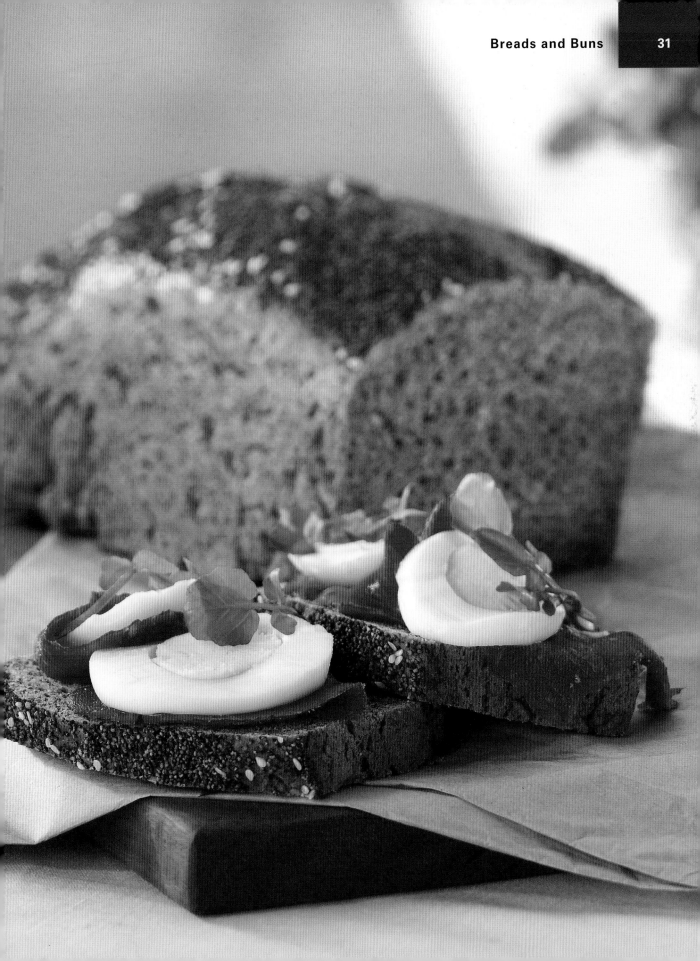

Fruit and Nut Bread

Makes 1 loaf

One of my fall and winter favourites. This bread provides the lightness of a white bread with the crunch of nuts, seeds and dried fruits with a hint of spice.

¼ cup (60 mL) warm water

1 Tbsp (15 mL) active dry yeast

2 tsp (10 mL) sugar

1 ½ cups (375 mL) tapioca starch

1 ½ cups (375 mL) white rice flour

½ cup (125 mL) chopped dates, soaked for a few minutes

½ cup (125 mL) chopped pecans

½ cup (125 mL) currants, soaked for a few minutes

¼ cup (60 mL) chopped pumpkin seeds

¼ cup (60 mL) milk powder

2 Tbsp (30 mL) pea fibre 80

2 Tbsp (30 mL) poppy seeds

4 tsp (20 mL) sugar

1 Tbsp (15 mL) xanthan gum

1 tsp (5 mL) allspice

1 tsp (5 mL) cinnamon (optional)

1 tsp (5 mL) dough improver (see page 19)

1 tsp (5 mL) salt

1 cup (250 mL) water

2 large eggs, room temperature (see page 6)

¼ cup (60 mL) oil

2 Tbsp (30 mL) egg whites, room temperature

2 Tbsp (30 mL) honey

1 tsp (5 mL) vanilla

Place first 3 ingredients in a small bowl. Let stand for 10 minutes until foamy.

Thoroughly mix next 15 ingredients in an extra-large bowl.

Blend last 6 ingredients in a separate bowl. Add egg mixture and yeast mixture to flour mixture. Mix until a smooth batter is formed. Pour batter into a greased 9 x 5 inch (23 x 12.5 cm) baking pan and smooth with a wet spatula. Place in a warm place and cover with a damp towel. Let rise until doubled in size. Place pan in a 350°F (175°C) oven on middle rack. Bake for 50 minutes until bread sounds hollow when tapped on bottom. Place pan on a wire rack to cool.

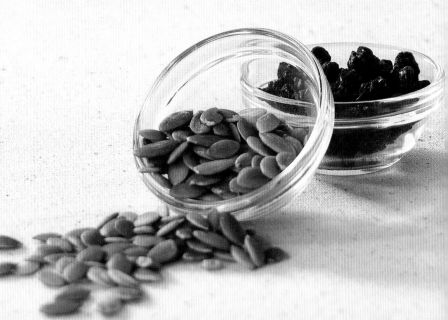

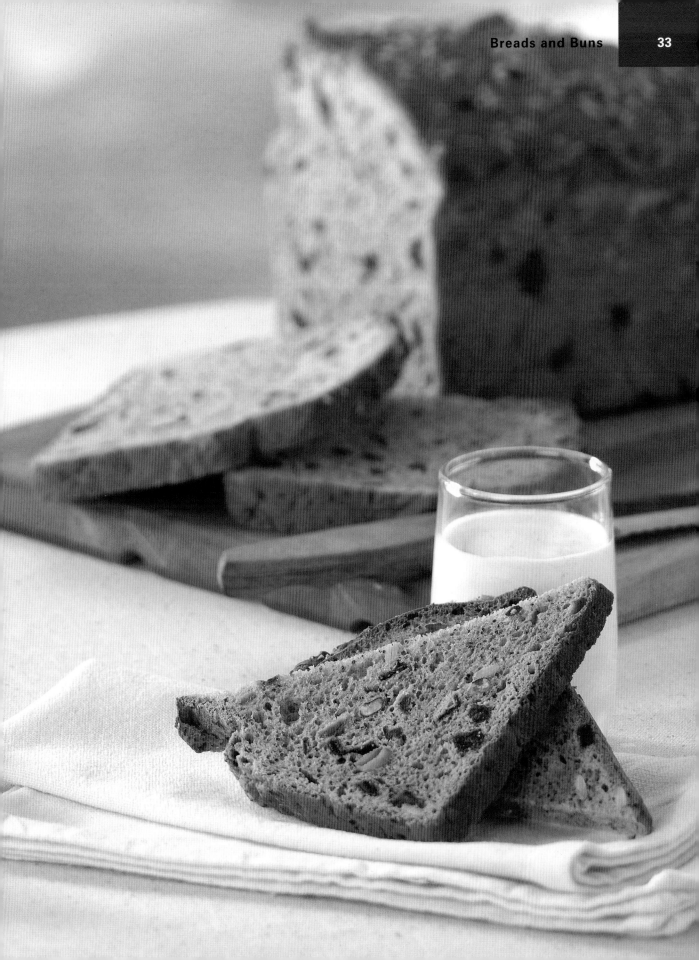

Festive Bread

Makes 1 loaf

A colourful and bright addition to the holiday season. Spread with real butter, this bread is a sweet morning delight.

¼ cup (60 mL) warm water

1 Tbsp (15 mL) active dry yeast

2 tsp (10 mL) sugar

1 ½ cups (375 mL) white rice flour

1 cup (250 mL) tapioca starch

¾ cup (175 mL) glazed fruit mix

½ cup (125 mL) pea starch

⅓ cup (75 mL) chopped glazed green cherries

⅓ cup (75 mL) chopped glazed red cherries

¼ cup (60 mL) milk powder

2 Tbsp (30 mL) pea fibre 80

4 tsp (20 mL) sugar

1 Tbsp (15 mL) xanthan gum

1 ¼ tsp (6 mL) pumpkin spice

1 tsp (5 mL) dough improver (see page 19)

1 tsp (5 mL) salt

1 cup (250 mL) water

¼ cup (60 mL) oil

2 large eggs, room temperature (see page 6)

2 Tbsp (30 mL) egg whites, room temperature

2 Tbsp (30 mL) honey

1 tsp (5 mL) vanilla

Place first 3 ingredients in a small bowl. Let stand for 10 minutes until foamy.

Thoroughly mix next 13 ingredients in an extra-large bowl.

Blend last 6 ingredients in a separate bowl. Add egg mixture and yeast mixture to flour mixture. Mix until a smooth batter is formed. Pour batter into a greased 9 x 5 inch (23 x 12.5 cm) baking pan and smooth with a wet spatula. Place in a warm place and cover with a damp towel. Let rise until doubled in size. Place pan in a 350°F (175°C) oven on middle rack. Bake for 50 minutes until bread sounds hollow when tapped on bottom. Place pan on a wire rack to cool.

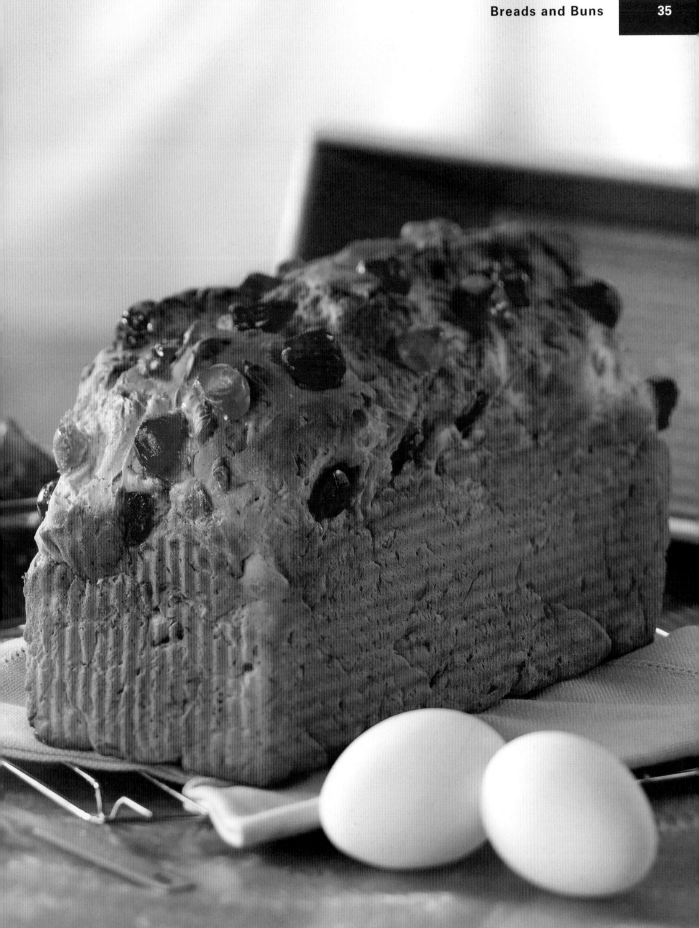

Cinnamon Raisin Bread

Makes 1 loaf

With plump raisins galore and the fragrance of cinnamon, this yummy bread will satisfy even the sweetest tooth.

¼ cup (60 mL) warm water

1 Tbsp (15 mL) active dry yeast

2 tsp (10 mL) sugar

1 ½ cups (375 mL) tapioca starch

1 ½ cups (375 mL) Thompson raisins

1 ½ cups (375 mL) white rice flour

¼ cup (60 mL) milk powder

2 Tbsp (30 mL) pea fibre 80

4 tsp (20 mL) sugar

1 Tbsp (15 mL) xanthan gum

1 tsp (5 mL) cinnamon (optional)

1 tsp (5 mL) dough improver (see page 19)

1 tsp (5 mL) salt

1 cup (250 mL) water

2 large eggs, room temperature (see page 6)

¼ cup (60 mL) oil

2 Tbsp (30 mL) egg whites, room temperature

2 Tbsp (30 mL) honey

1 tsp (5 mL) vanilla

Place first 3 ingredients in a small bowl. Let stand for 10 minutes until foamy.

Thoroughly mix next 10 ingredients in an extra-large bowl.

Blend last 6 ingredients in a separate bowl. Add egg mixture and yeast mixture to flour mixture. Mix until a smooth batter is formed. Pour into a greased 9 x 5 inch (23 x 12.5 cm) baking pan and smooth with a wet spatula. Place in a warm place and cover with a damp towel. Let rise until doubled in size. Place pans in a 350°F (175°C) oven on middle rack. Bake for 55 minutes until bread sounds hollow when tapped on bottom. Place pans on a wire rack to cool.

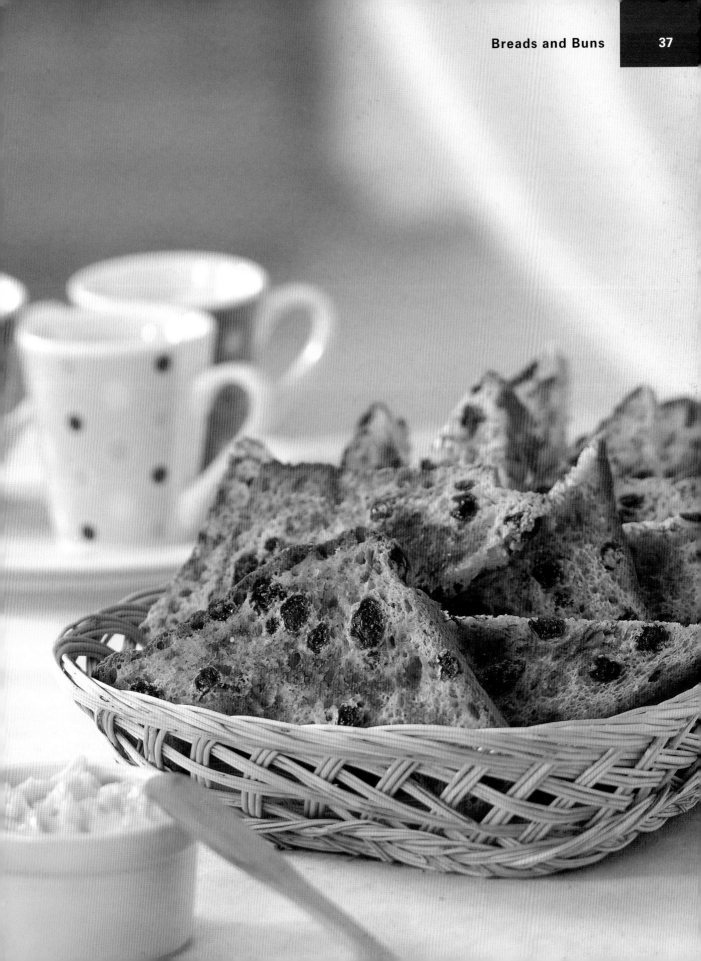

Good Morning Rolls

Makes 12

A typical breakfast bun in Germany. Don't save these just for Sunday morning.

¼ cup (60 mL) warm water

1 Tbsp (15 mL) active dry yeast

2 tsp (10 mL) sugar

1 ½ cups (375 mL) tapioca starch

1 cup (250 mL) sultanas, soaked for a few minutes

1 cup (250 mL) white rice flour

½ cup (125 mL) sweet rice flour

¼ cup (60 mL) milk powder

7 tsp (35 mL) sugar

1 Tbsp (15 mL) xanthan gum

1 ½ tsp (7 mL) baking powder

1 tsp (5 mL) baking soda

1 tsp (5 mL) dough improver (see page 19)

1 tsp (5 mL) salt

1 cup (250 mL) water

2 large eggs, room temperature (see page 6)

¼ cup (60 mL) oil

2 Tbsp (30 mL) egg whites, room temperature

2 Tbsp (30 mL) honey

1 tsp (5 mL) vanilla

Place first 3 ingredients in a small bowl. Let stand for 10 minutes until foamy.

Thoroughly mix next 11 ingredients in an extra-large bowl.

Blend next 6 ingredients in a separate bowl. Add egg mixture and yeast mixture to flour mixture. Mix until a smooth batter is formed. Drop dough onto a greased baking sheet with an ice cream scoop (#20 or about ¼ cup [60 mL]). Smooth with a wet spatula. Place in a warm place and cover with a damp towel. Let rise until doubled in size. Place pan in a 350°F (175°C) oven on middle rack. Bake for 25 to 30 minutes until browned. Place pan on a wire rack to cool.

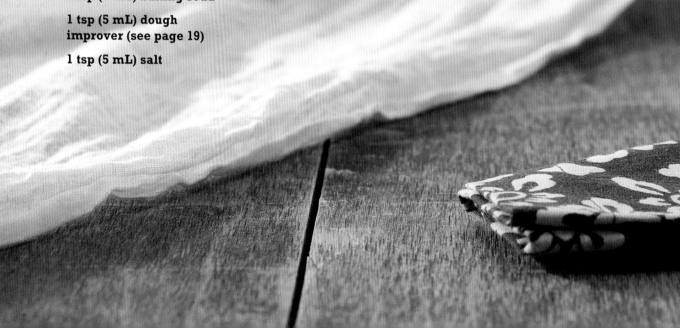

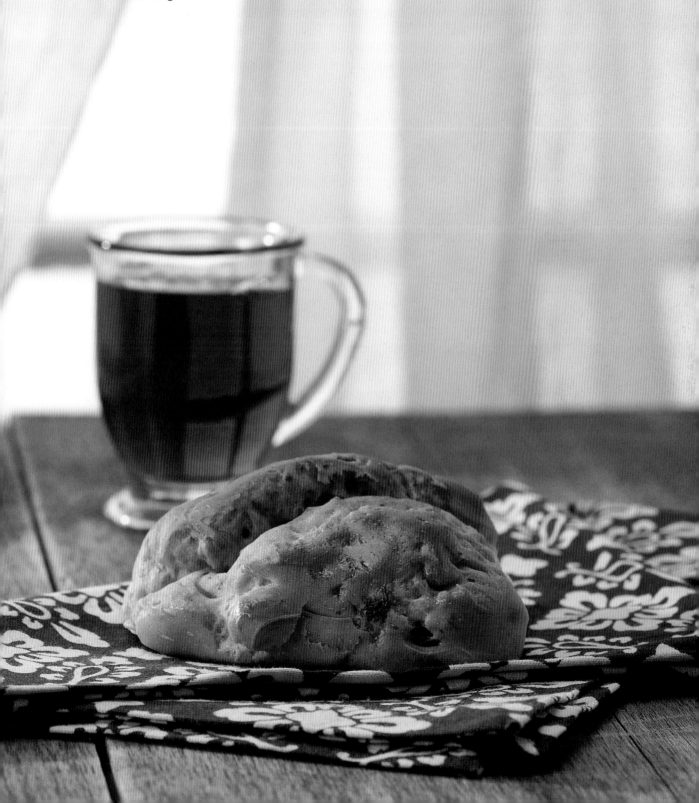

Adding honey to gluten-free baked goods keeps them softer for longer.

Milk Buns

Makes 12

Crusty outside and chewy inside, these nice buns are topped with poppy seeds. Serve with some butter and a bit of jam.

¼ cup (60 mL) warm water

1 Tbsp (15 mL) active dry yeast

2 tsp (10 mL) sugar

1 ½ cups (375 mL) tapioca starch

1 cup (250 mL) white rice flour

½ cup (125 mL) pea starch

¼ cup (60 mL) whey powder

4 tsp (20 mL) sugar

1 Tbsp (15 mL) xanthan gum

1 tsp (5 mL) dough improver (see page 19)

1 tsp (5 mL) salt

1 cup (250 mL) hot milk

2 large eggs, room temperature (see page 6)

¼ cup (60 mL) oil

2 Tbsp (30 mL) egg whites, room temperature

2 Tbsp (30 mL) honey

Egg Wash

1 large egg, room temperature (see page 6)

1 Tbsp (15 mL) milk

¼ cup (60 mL) poppy seeds

Place first 3 ingredients in a small bowl. Let stand for 10 minutes until foamy.

Thoroughly mix next 8 ingredients in an extra-large bowl.

Blend next 5 ingredients in a separate bowl. Mix until a smooth batter is formed. Drop dough onto a greased baking sheet with an ice cream scoop (#20 or about ¼ cup [60 mL]). Smooth with a wet spatula.

Beat third egg in a small bowl and add milk. Brush over batter.

Top with poppy seeds. Place in a warm place and cover with a damp towel. Let rise until doubled in size. Place pan in a 350°F (175°C) oven on middle rack. Bake for 25 to 30 minutes until browned. Place pan on a wire rack to cool.

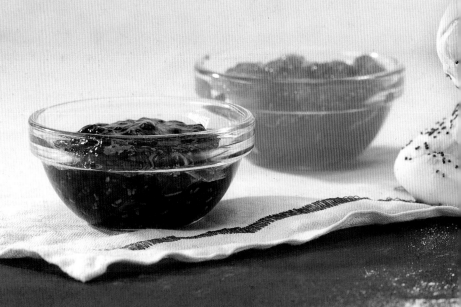

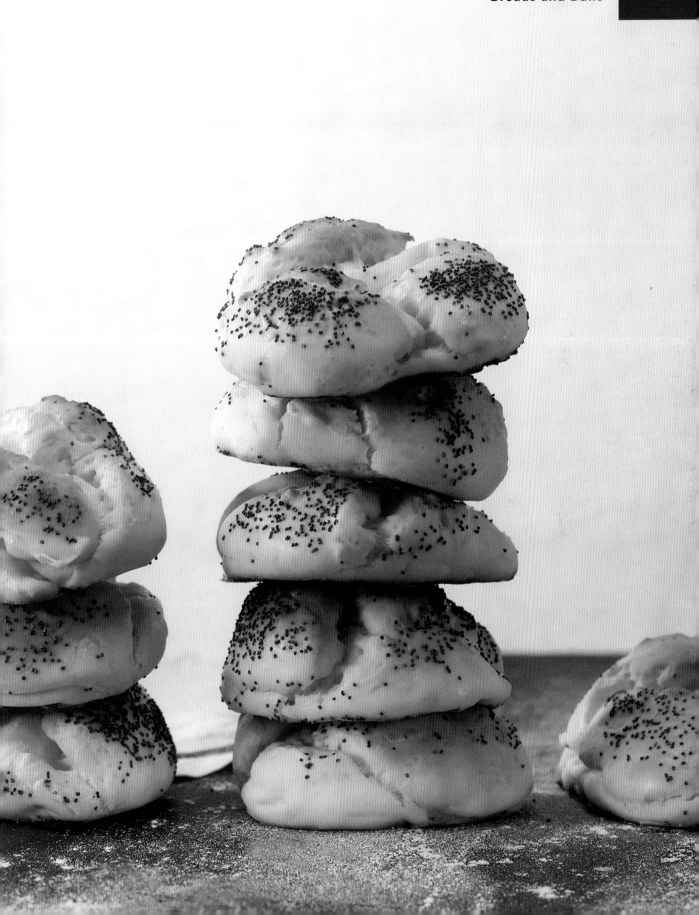

Fibre Buns

Makes 12

A good balance of softness and fibre content makes this a great everyday bun. Provides about 3 g fibre per bun.

¼ cup (60 mL) warm water

1 Tbsp (15 mL) active dry yeast

2 tsp (10 mL) sugar

1 cup (250 mL) brown rice flour

¾ cup (175 mL) tapioca starch

½ cup (125 mL) pea starch

½ cup (125 mL) sorghum flour

¼ cup (60 mL) whey powder

4 mL (20 mL) sugar

1 Tbsp (15 mL) pea fibre III

1 Tbsp (15 mL) pea fibre 80

1 Tbsp (15 mL) xanthan gum

2 tsp (10 mL) baking powder

1 tsp (5 mL) dough improver (see page 19)

1 tsp (5 mL) salt

1 ¼ cups (300 mL) water

2 large eggs, room temperature (see page 6)

¼ cup (60 mL) oil

2 Tbsp (30 mL) egg whites, room temperature

2 Tbsp (30 mL) honey

Place first 3 ingredients in a small bowl. Let stand for 10 minutes until foamy.

Thoroughly mix next 12 ingredients in an extra-large bowl.

Blend last 5 ingredients in a separate bowl. Add egg mixture and yeast mixture to flour mixture. Mix until a smooth batter is formed. Drop dough onto a greased baking sheet with an ice cream scoop (#20 or about ¼ cup [60 mL]). Smooth with a wet spatula. Place in a warm place and cover with a damp towel. Let rise until about doubled in size. Place pan in a 350°F (175°C) oven on middle rack. Bake for 25 to 30 minutes until browned. Place pan on a wire rack to cool.

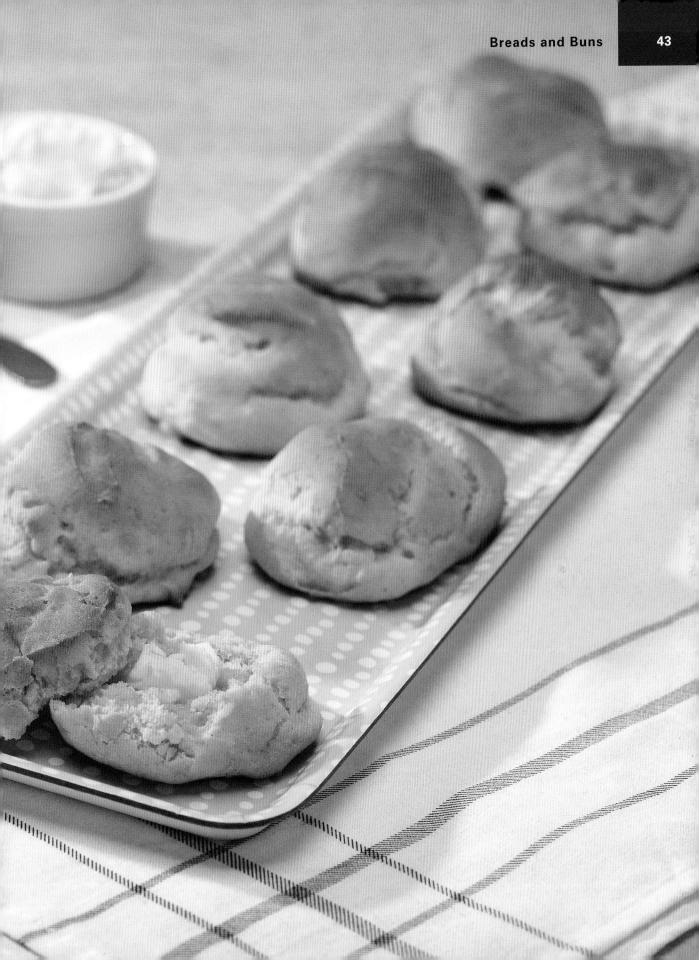

Flax and Sun Buns

Makes 12

A very attractive whole grain–style bun with the goodness of flax and sunflower seeds.

¼ cup (60 mL) warm water

1 Tbsp (15 mL) active dry yeast

2 tsp (10 mL) sugar

1 cup (250 mL) brown rice flour

¾ cup (175 mL) tapioca starch

½ cup (125 mL) flaxseed

½ cup (125 mL) pea starch

½ cup (125 mL) sorghum flour

½ cup (125 mL) sunflower seeds

¼ cup (60 mL) whey powder

4 tsp (20 mL) sugar

1 Tbsp (15 mL) pea fibre III

1 Tbsp (15 mL) pea fibre 80

1 Tbsp (15 mL) xanthan gum

2 tsp (10 mL) baking powder

1 tsp (5 mL) dough improver (see page 19)

1 tsp (5 mL) salt

1 ¼ cups (300 mL) water

2 large eggs, room temperature (see page 6)

¼ cup (60 mL) oil

2 Tbsp (30 mL) egg whites, room temperature

2 Tbsp (30 mL) honey

Egg Wash

1 large egg, room temperature (see page 6)

2 Tbsp (30 mL) milk

flaxseed or sunflower seeds, for topping

Place first 3 ingredients in a small bowl. Let stand for 10 minutes until foamy.

Thoroughly mix next 14 ingredients in an extra-large bowl.

Blend next 5 ingredients in a separate bowl. Add egg mixture and yeast mixture to flour mixture. Mix until a smooth batter is formed. Drop dough onto a greased baking sheet with an ice cream scoop (#20 or about ¼ cup [60 mL]). Smooth with a wet spatula.

Beat third egg in a small bowl and add milk. Brush over batter.

Top with seeds. Place in a warm place and cover with a damp towel. Let rise until doubled in size. Place pan in a 350°F (175°C) oven on middle rack. Bake for 25 to 30 minutes until browned. Place pan on a wire rack to cool.

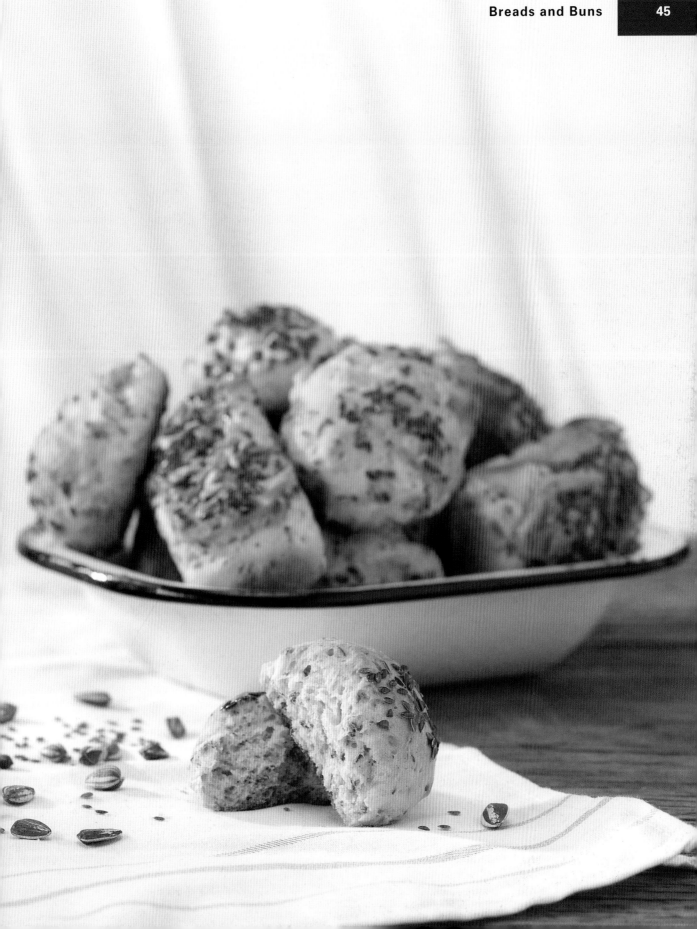

Hamburger and Hot Dog Buns

Makes 12

A light, airy bun that's perfect for your favourite patty, hot dog or sausage. I've made hamburger buns here, but you can make whatever type of buns you'd like. Just adjust the batter amount in the pan to the desired thickness and shape of bun.

¼ cup (60 mL) warm water

1 Tbsp (15 mL) active dry yeast

2 tsp (10 mL) sugar

¾ cup (175 mL) pea starch

¾ cup (175 mL) tapioca starch

½ cup (125 mL) cornstarch

¼ cup (60 mL) whey powder

1 Tbsp (15 mL) pea fibre 80

2 tsp (10 mL) baking powder

2 tsp (10 mL) xanthan gum

1 tsp (5 mL) dough improver (see page 19)

1 tsp (5 mL) salt

1 tsp (5 mL) sugar

1 cup (250 mL) water

¼ cup (60 mL) oil

2 Tbsp (30 mL) egg whites, room temperature

Place first 3 ingredients in a small bowl. Let stand for 10 minutes until foamy.

Thoroughly mix next 10 ingredients in an extra-large bowl.

Blend last 3 ingredients in a separate bowl. Add egg white mixture and yeast mixture to flour mixture. Mix until a smooth batter is formed. Pour batter about ¼ to ½ inch (6 to 12 mm) high in greased bun pans. If you don't have bun pans, you can shape some with folded-over foil shaped into bun forms. Place in a warm place and cover with a damp towel. Let rise until increased by about 50% in size. Place pans in a 350°F (175°C) oven on middle rack. Bake for 25 to 30 minutes until browned. Remove pans from oven. Place buns upside down on a wire rack to cool. Serve with your favourite toppings.

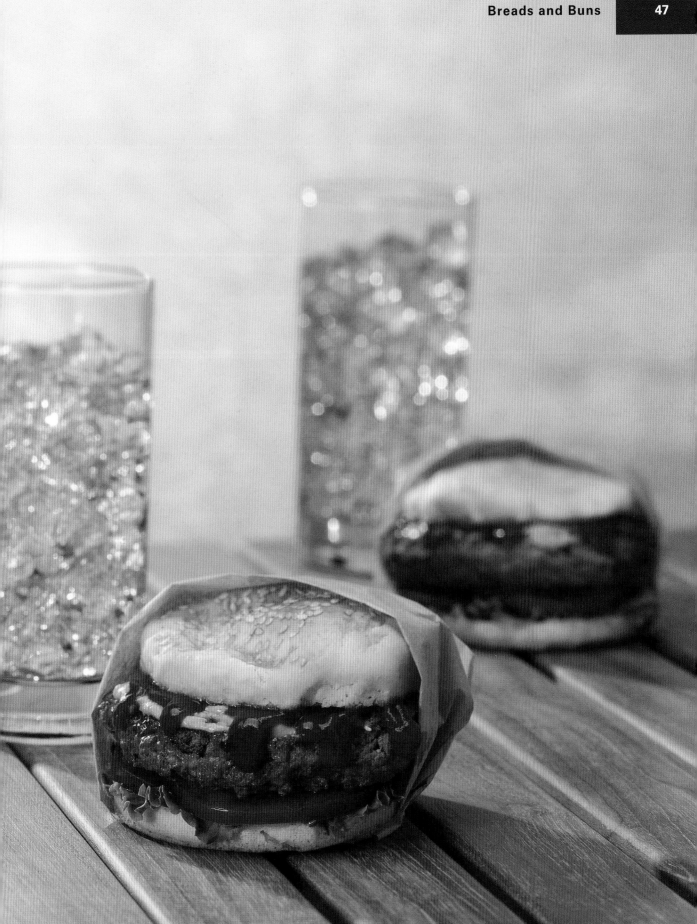

Cinnamon Buns

Makes 12

Yummy, sweet, gooey, mouthwatering. Always eat these cinnamon buns while still warm and don't just eat one.

½ cup (125 mL) warm water

1 Tbsp (15 mL) active dry yeast

1 Tbsp (15 mL) sugar

1 ½ cups (375 mL) tapioca starch

1 cup (250 mL) white rice flour

½ cup (125 mL) pea starch

¼ cup (60 mL) milk powder

2 Tbsp (30 mL) xanthan gum

1 Tbsp (15 mL) sugar

1 tsp (5 mL) dough improver (see page 19)

1 tsp (5 mL) salt

½ cup (125 mL) water

¼ cup (60 mL) oil

2 large eggs, room temperature (see page 6)

2 Tbsp (30 mL) egg whites, room temperature

2 Tbsp (30 mL) honey

2 Tbsp (30 mL) butter, melted

1 cup (250 mL) brown sugar

1 Tbsp (15 mL) cinnamon

Egg Wash
1 large egg, room temperature (see page 6)

1 Tbsp (15 mL) milk

½ cup (125 mL) butter, melted

1 tsp (5 mL) sweet rice flour

Place first 3 ingredients in a small bowl. Let stand for 10 minutes until foamy.

Thoroughly mix next 8 ingredients in an extra-large bowl.

Blend next 5 ingredients in a separate bowl. Mix until a smooth dough is formed. Turn out dough onto surface lightly floured with sweet rice flour. Roll out to rectangular shape (about 9 x 16 inches [23 x 40 cm]). Brush with first amount of melted butter.

Mix brown sugar and cinnamon in a small bowl. Sprinkle half evenly over dough, leaving about 1 inch (2.5 cm) edge along side of closest long length.

Beat third egg in a small bowl and add milk. Brush egg wash over 1 inch (2.5 cm) edge of dough. Gently roll up dough from long edge farthest from you. Roll tightly but don't press too hard.

Blend second amount of butter, sweet rice flour and remaining brown sugar mixture. Spread into 9 x 13 inch (23 x 33 cm) baking pan. Cut roll into 1 inch (2.5 cm) slices. Place side by side in baking pan. Brush each roll with egg wash. Place in a warm place and cover with a damp towel. Let rise until doubled in size. Place pan in a 350°F (175°C) oven on middle rack. Bake for 25 to 30 minutes until browned. Remove pan from oven. Place buns upside down on a plate to cool.

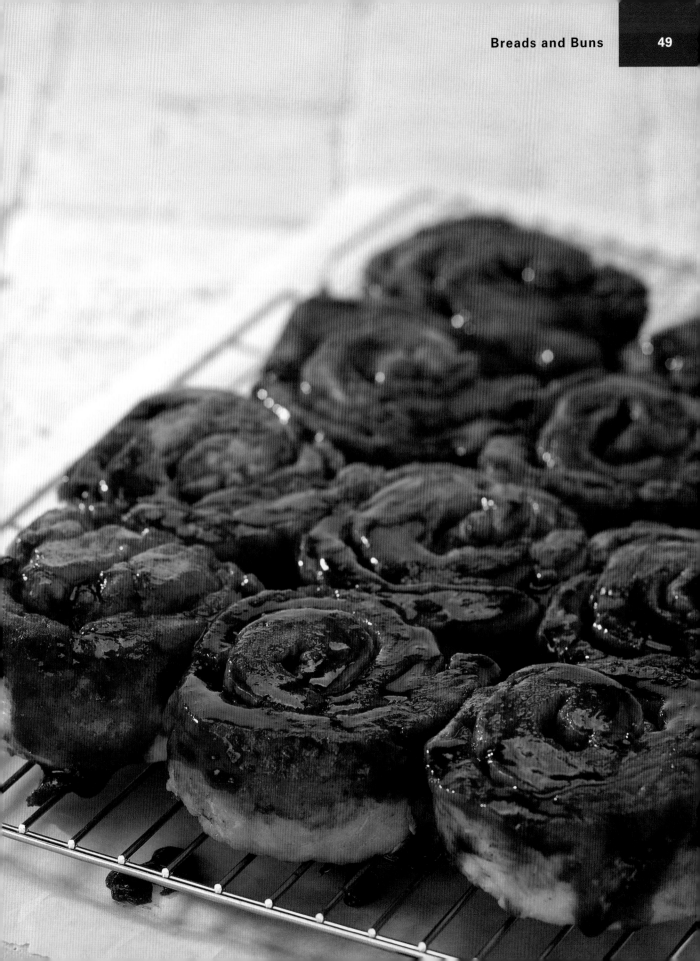

Hot Cross Buns

Makes 12

A bun with the classic taste, smell and look of the traditional Easter favourites.

¼ cup (60 mL) warm water

1 Tbsp (15 mL) active dry yeast

2 tsp (10 mL) sugar

Cross Icing

1 cup (250 mL) icing sugar

1 Tbsp (15 mL) butter

2 Tbsp (30 mL) lemon juice (approximately)

Glaze

½ cup (125 mL) apricot jam

2 Tbsp (30 mL) hot water

1 ½ cups (375 mL) white rice flour

1 cup (250 mL) tapioca starch

½ cup (125 mL) currants, soaked for a few minutes

½ cup (125 mL) glazed fruit mix

½ cup (125 mL) sweet rice flour

¼ cup (60 mL) milk powder

7 tsp (35 mL) sugar

1 Tbsp (15 mL) xanthan gum

1 ½ tsp (7 mL) baking powder

1 ½ tsp (7 mL) pumpkin spice

1 tsp (5 mL) baking soda

1 tsp (5 mL) dough improver (see page 19)

1 tsp (5 mL) salt

1 ¼ cups (300 mL) water

2 large eggs, room temperature (see page 6)

¼ cup (60 mL) oil

2 Tbsp (30 mL) egg whites, room temperature

2 Tbsp (30 mL) honey

Place first 3 ingredients in a small bowl. Let stand for 10 minutes until foamy.

Mix icing sugar and butter in a small bowl. Add lemon juice as needed until mixture is a pouring consistency. Set aside.

Heat apricot jam and water. Place mixture in sieve. Discard solids; reserve and set aside clear liquid.

Thoroughly mix next 13 ingredients in an extra-large bowl.

(continued on next page)

Blend last 5 ingredients in a separate bowl. Add egg
mixture and yeast mixture to flour mixture. Mix until a
smooth batter is formed. Scoop batter into a 9 x 13 inch
(23 x 33 cm) baking pan and smooth top with a wet spatula.
Place in a warm place and cover with a damp towel. Let rise
until doubled in size. Place pan in a 350°F (175°C) oven on
middle rack. Bake for 50 minutes until browned. Place pan
on a wire rack to cool. Once completely cooled, brush buns
with glaze, then pipe a cross with icing onto each bun.

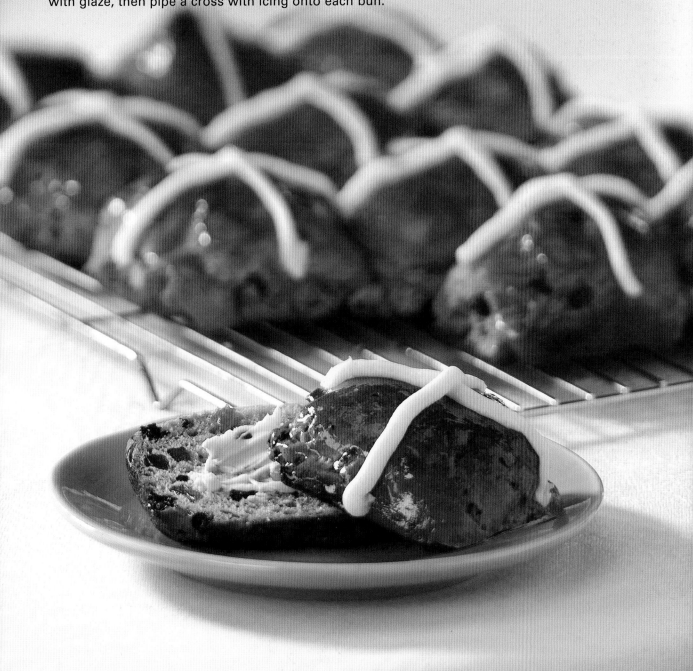

New York Bagels

Makes 8 to 10

A nice bagel prepared in the New York way. This bagel goes with everything, from simple cream cheese to a full works sandwich filling. Bagels take a little bit more effort than other buns, but they're worth it.

¼ cup (60 mL) warm water

1 ½ Tbsp (25 mL) active dry yeast

2 tsp (10 mL) sugar

1 ¼ cups (300 mL) tapioca starch

1 ¼ cups (300 mL) white rice flour

½ cup (125 mL) sweet rice flour

¼ cup (60 mL) whey powder

2 Tbsp (30 mL) pea fibre 80

1 Tbsp (15 mL) sugar

4 tsp (20 mL) xanthan gum

1 tsp (5 mL) dough improver (see page 19)

¾ tsp (4 mL) salt

1 ¼ cups (300 mL) water

1 large egg, room temperature (see page 6)

2 Tbsp (30 mL) egg whites, room temperature

Egg Wash

1 large egg, room temperature (see page 6)

1 Tbsp (15 mL) milk

Place first 3 ingredients in a small bowl. Let stand for 10 minutes until foamy.

Thoroughly mix next 9 ingredients in an extra-large bowl.

Blend next 3 ingredients in a separate bowl. Add egg mixture and yeast mixture to flour mixture. Mix until a smooth dough is formed. Turn out dough onto surface lightly floured with white rice flour. Roll out dough into long strands ¾ to 1 inch (2 to 2.5 cm) thick. Cut each into 6 to 8 inch (15 to 20 cm) pieces. Form each piece into circles, pinching dough ends together. Place in a warm place and cover with a damp towel. Let rise until doubled in size. Meanwhile, bring a large pot of water to a rolling boil. Place proofed bagels into boiling water for 30 to 45 seconds. (Alternatively, bagels can be baked in an oven with steam injection for the first 60 seconds of the bake cycle. The boiling step can be skipped in this case.) Remove from water and place on paper towels to dry. Place bagels on greased baking sheets.

Beat second egg in a small bowl and add milk. Brush egg wash on bagels. Place an ovenproof bowl of hot water in the oven. Bake bagels in a 425°F (220°C) oven on middle rack for 15 to 20 minutes. Place pans on wire racks to cool.

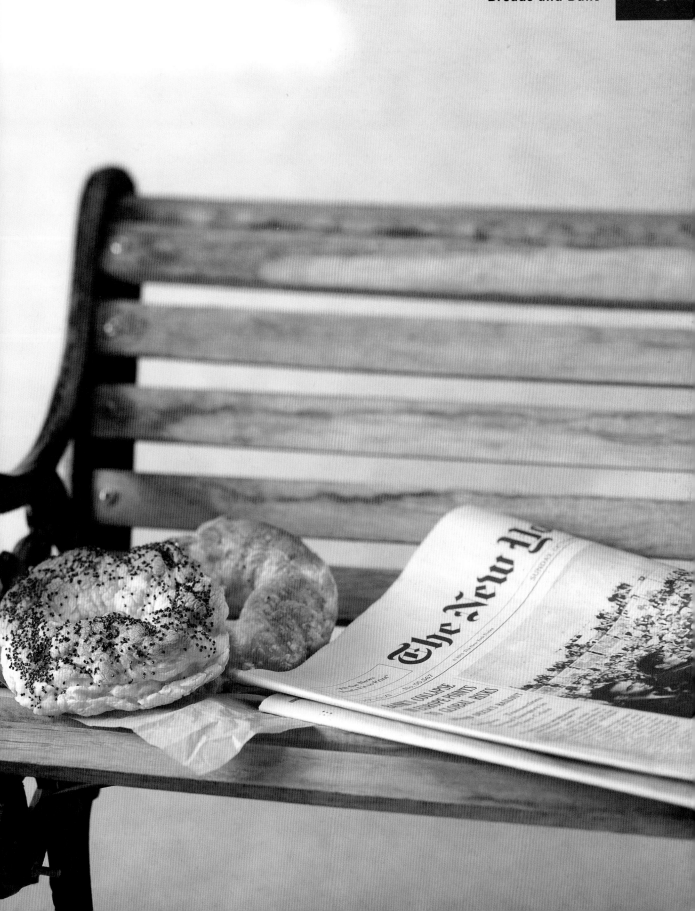

Cinnamon Raisin Bagels

Makes 8 to 10

A simple dap of soft butter or plain cream cheese is the perfect companion for this aromatic, slightly sweet bagel. Add a hot, foamy latte and you'll feel like you've been transported to the French Riviera.

¼ cup (60 mL) warm water

1 ½ Tbsp (25 mL) active dry yeast

2 tsp (10 mL) sugar

1 ¼ cups (300 mL) tapioca starch

1 ¼ cups (300 mL) white rice flour

¾ cup (175 mL) coarsely chopped raisins

½ cup (125 mL) sweet rice flour

¼ cup (60 mL) whey powder

2 Tbsp (30 mL) pea fibre 80

1 ½ Tbsp (25 mL) sugar

1 Tbsp (15 mL) xanthan gum

1 tsp (5 mL) cinnamon

1 tsp (5 mL) dough improver (see page 19)

¾ tsp (4 mL) salt

1 cup (250 mL) water

1 large egg, room temperature (see page 6)

2 Tbsp (30 mL) egg whites, room temperature

Egg Wash

1 large egg, room temperature (see page 6)

1 Tbsp (15 mL) milk

Place first 3 ingredients in a small bowl. Let stand for 10 minutes until foamy.

Thoroughly mix next 11 ingredients in an extra-large bowl.

Blend next 3 ingredients in a separate bowl. Add egg mixture and yeast mixture to flour mixture. Mix until a smooth dough is formed. Turn out dough onto surface lightly floured with white rice flour. Roll out dough into long strands ¾ to 1 inch (2 to 2.5 cm) thick. Cut each into 6 to 8 inch (15 to 20 cm) pieces. Form each piece into circles, pinching dough ends together. Place in a warm place and cover with a damp towel. Let rise until doubled in size. Meanwhile, bring a large pot of water to a rolling boil. Place proofed bagels into boiling water for 30 to 45 seconds. (Alternatively, bagels can be baked in an oven with steam injection for the first 60 seconds of the bake cycle. The boiling step can be skipped in this case.) Remove from water and place on paper towels to dry. Place bagels on greased baking pans.

Beat second egg in a small bowl and add milk. Brush egg wash on bagels. Place an ovenproof bowl of hot water in the oven. Bake bagels in a 425°F (220°C) oven on middle rack for 15 to 20 minutes. Place pans on wire racks to cool.

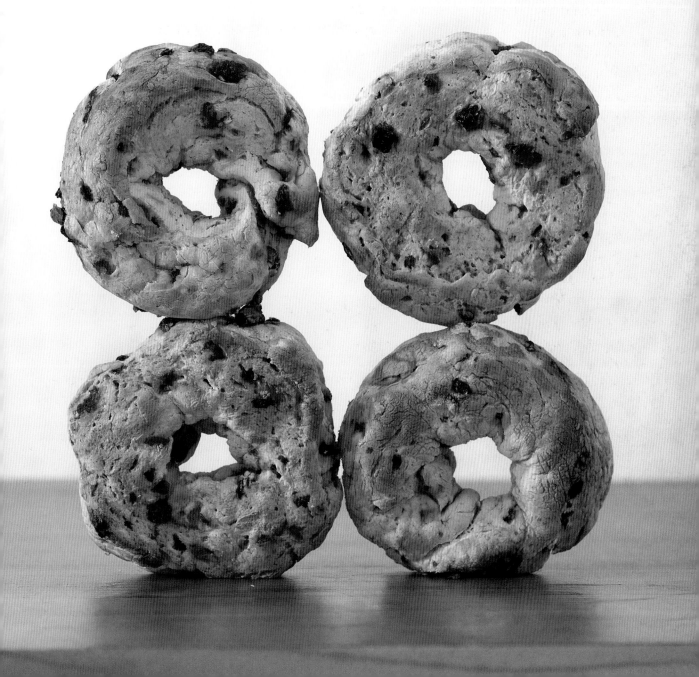

Basic Pizza Crust

Makes 2

A basic pizza crust that's chewy and perfect for your favourite toppings. You can spread out the dough by hand or, if handled carefully, roll it out, provided you use sweet rice flour for dusting. The pizza crust recipe does not include any herbs or flavouring, but those could be added to taste. I prefer a regular crust with the flavouring supplied by the toppings and sauce.

½ cup (125 mL) warm water

1 Tbsp (15 mL) pizza crust yeast

2 tsp (10 mL) sugar

1 ½ cups (375 mL) tapioca starch

1 cup (250 mL) white rice flour

½ cup (125 mL) sweet rice flour

¼ cup (60 mL) whey powder

2 Tbsp (30 mL) pea fibre 80

2 Tbsp (30 mL) sugar

4 tsp (20 mL) xanthan gum

1 tsp (5 mL) dough improver (see page 19)

1 tsp (5 mL) salt

1 ¼ cups (300 mL) water

½ cup (125 mL) egg whites, room temperature

3 Tbsp (45 mL) oil

2 Tbsp (30 mL) fine cornmeal

pizza toppings as desired

Place first 3 ingredients in a small bowl. Let stand for 10 minutes until foamy.

Thoroughly mix next 9 ingredients in an extra-large bowl.

Blend next 3 ingredients in a separate bowl. Add egg white mixture and yeast mixture to flour mixture. The dough will look like thick cake batter.

Dust two 12 inch (30 cm) pizza pans with cornmeal. Divide dough equally onto pizza pans, and spread and smooth with a wet spatula. Place in a warm place and cover with a damp towel. Let rise until doubled in size. Place pans in a 350°F (175°C) oven on middle rack. Bake for about 10 minutes. Remove pans from oven. Add desired pizza toppings. Bake for about 10 minutes until desired browning.

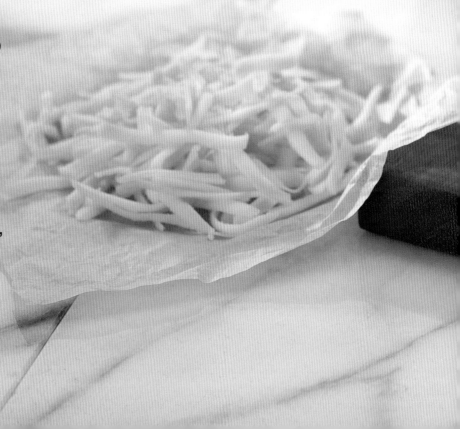

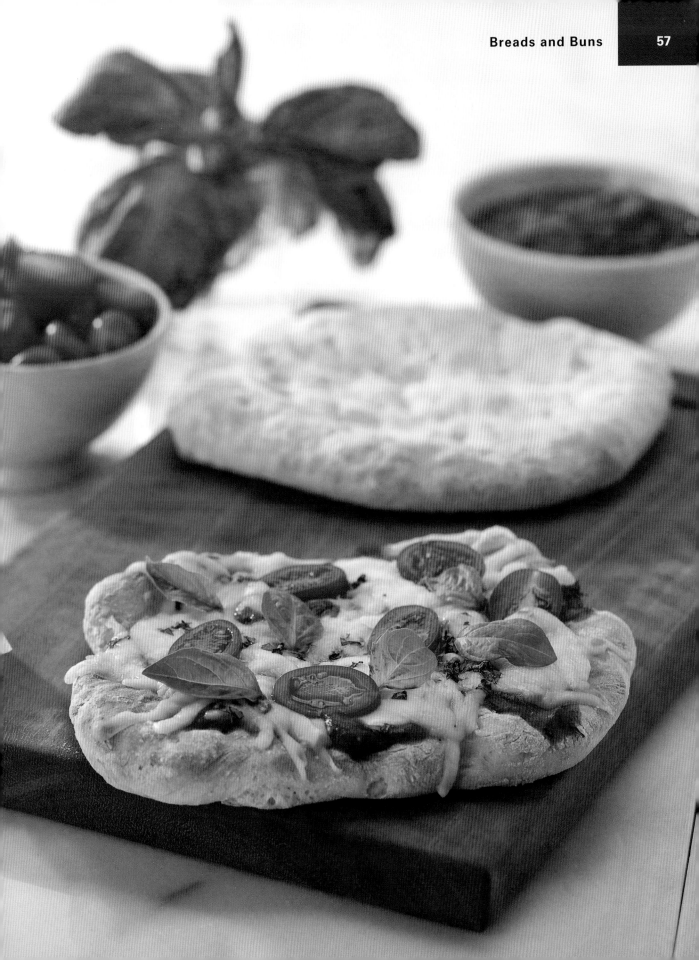

Thin Pizza Crust

Makes 2

A thicker dough that you can stretch to roll out a thin pizza crust, if you prefer more topping than crust. I also use this recipe for pizza pockets.

⅔ cup (150 mL) sweet rice flour

⅔ cup (150 mL) tapioca starch

⅓ cup (75 mL) pea starch

2 Tbsp (30 mL) sugar

2 Tbsp (30 mL) whey powder

1 ½ Tbsp (25 mL) pea fibre III

1 ½ Tbsp (25 mL) yeast

2 tsp (10 mL) xanthan gum

1 ¼ tsp (6 mL) guar gum

¼ tsp (1 mL) salt

½ cup (125 mL) water

3 Tbsp (45 mL) oil

2 Tbsp (30 mL) egg whites, room temperature

1 large egg, room temperature (see page 6)

pizza toppings as desired

Preheat oven to 400°F (200°C). Mix first 10 ingredients in a medium metal bowl.

Blend next 4 ingredients in a separate bowl. Add egg mixture to flour mixture. Knead together or use a heavy-duty mixer (such as a KitchenAid) with a dough hook attachment. Turn out dough onto surface lightly floured with sweet rice flour. Divide dough into 2 balls. Roll dough pieces out to desired thickness. Place on two 12 inch (30 cm) pizza pans and prick with a fork. Bake in preheated oven for 8 to 10 minutes.

Remove pizzas from oven. Add desired pizza toppings. Reduce heat to 350°F (175°C) and bake for 20 to 25 minutes until desired browning.

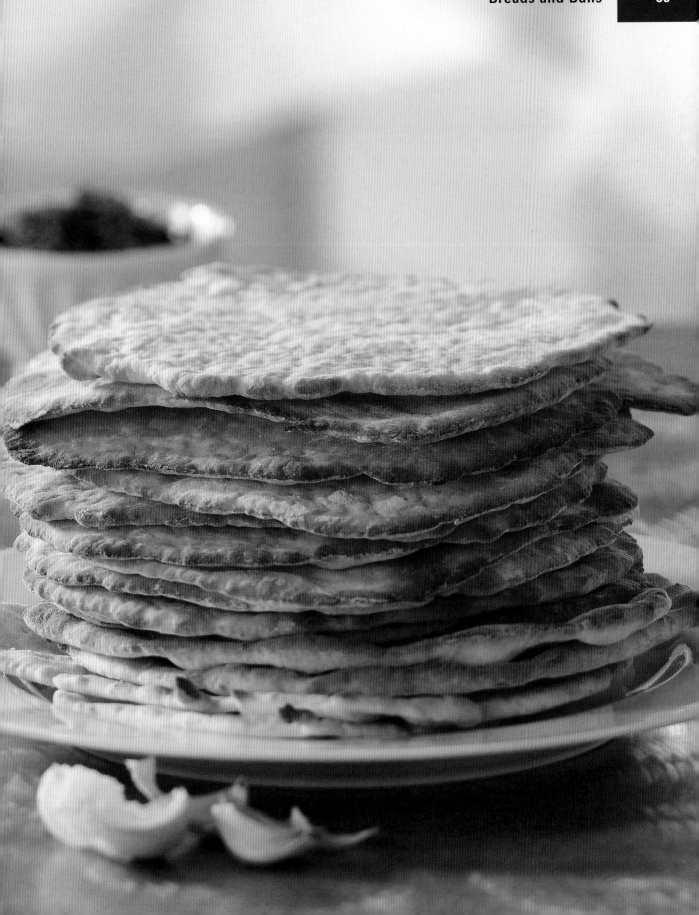

No-roll Easy Pizza Crust

Makes 2

This quick method for making a pizza crust doesn't involve rolling or heavy mixing. The recipe provides a batter-style dough for a pre-baked crust.

1 ⅛ cups (280 mL) pea starch

1 cup (250 mL) water

¾ cup (175 mL) tapioca starch

¼ cup (60 mL) whey powder

2 Tbsp (30 mL) egg whites, room temperature

2 Tbsp (30 mL) oil

1 Tbsp (15 mL) pea fibre 80

1 Tbsp (15 mL) sugar

2 tsp (10 mL) baking powder

2 tsp (10 mL) xanthan gum

2 tsp (10 mL) yeast

1 tsp (5 mL) dough improver (see page 19)

1 tsp (5 mL) salt

pizza toppings as desired

Preheat oven to 350°F (175°C). Blend first 13 ingredients in a heavy-duty mixer. Mix for 2 minutes. Spread pizza batter onto two lightly greased 10 inch (25 cm) pizza pans. Let rise for 10 minutes. Bake in preheated oven for 10 minutes.

Remove pizzas from oven. Add desired pizza toppings. Bake for 10 to 20 minutes until desired browning.

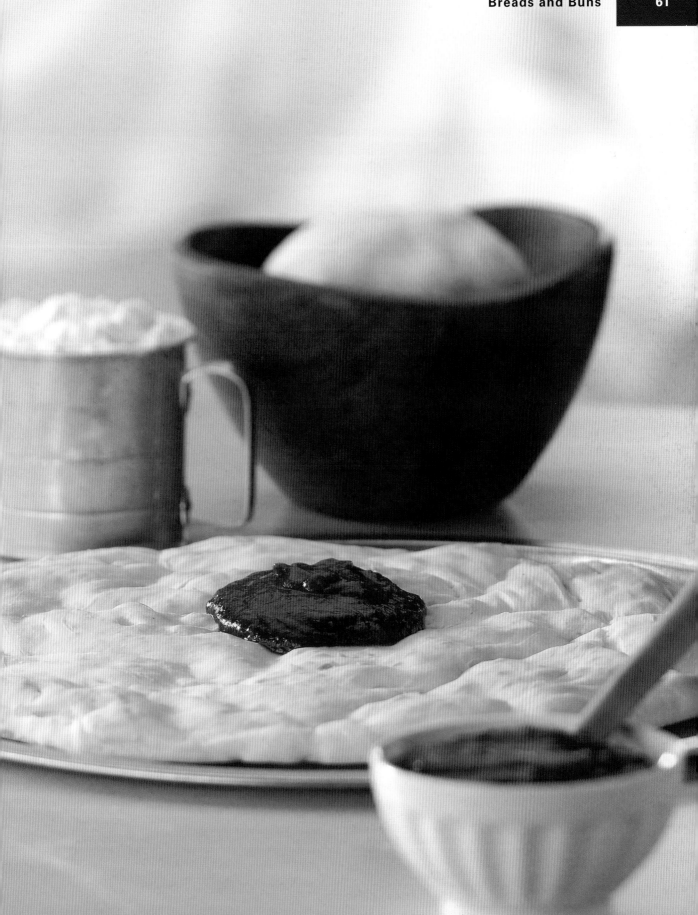

Banana Bread

Makes 1 loaf

Slice this flavourful staple into thick slices and take a bite into a rich, moist loaf. The overripe bananas provide just the right taste and look. I always add cinnamon.

1 cup (250 mL) sugar

½ cup (125 mL) brown rice flour

½ cup (125 mL) pea starch

½ cup (125 mL) sorghum flour

½ cup (125 mL) tapioca starch

2 tsp (10 mL) xanthan gum

1 tsp (5 mL) baking soda

1 tsp (5 mL) cinnamon (optional)

¼ tsp (1 mL) salt

4 large overripe bananas

2 large eggs, room temperature (see page 6), beaten

½ cup (125 mL) butter

1 tsp (5 mL) vanilla

Preheat oven to 350°F (175°C). Mix first 9 ingredients in an extra-large bowl.

Blend last 4 ingredients in a separate bowl. Fold banana mixture into flour mixture until all dry mixture is wet. Don't beat. Pour batter into a greased 8 x 4 inch (20 x 10 cm) baking pan. Bake in preheated oven for 50 minutes until wooden pick inserted in centre of loaf comes out clean. Place pan on a wire rack to cool.

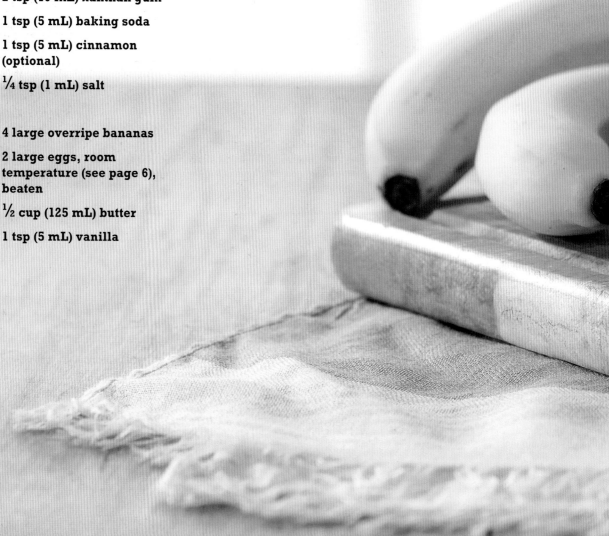

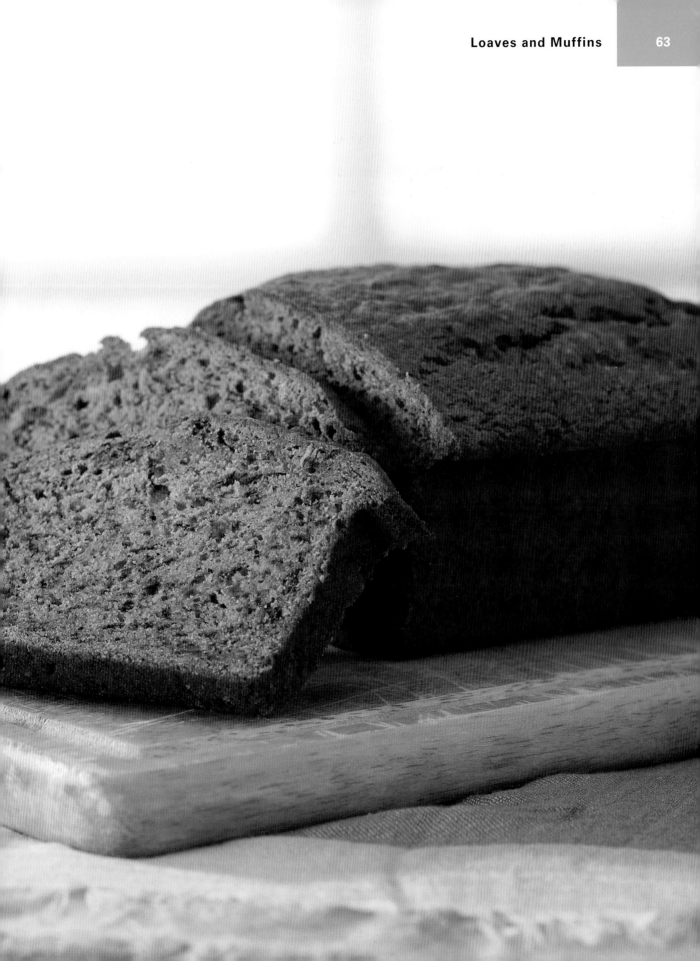

Nutty Carrot Loaf

Makes 1 loaf

A wonderful taste sensation of spices, carrot and nuts will lighten up your coffee time. This moist loaf is a filling snack anytime. Try drizzling the loaf with cream cheese icing (see page 95).

1 ½ cup (375 mL) sugar

1 cup (250 mL) golden raisins

⅔ cup (150 mL) chopped walnuts

½ cup (125 mL) brown rice flour

½ cup (125 mL) pea starch

½ cup (125 mL) sorghum flour

½ cup (125 mL) tapioca starch

2 tsp (10 mL) baking soda

2 tsp (10 mL) xanthan gum

1 tsp (5 mL) cinnamon

½ tsp (2 mL) nutmeg

½ tsp (2 mL) salt

4 large eggs, room temperature (see page 6), beaten

2 large carrots, finely grated

1 cup (250 mL) oil

½ cup (125 mL) crushed pineapple

1 tsp (5 mL) vanilla extract

Preheat oven to 350°F (175°C). Mix first 12 ingredients in an extra-large bowl.

Blend last 5 ingredients in a separate bowl. Fold carrot mixture into flour mixture until all dry mixture is wet. Don't beat. Pour batter into a greased 9 x 5 inch (23 x 12.5 cm) baking pan. Bake in preheated oven for 50 minutes until wooden pick inserted in centre of loaf comes out clean. Place pan on a wire rack to cool.

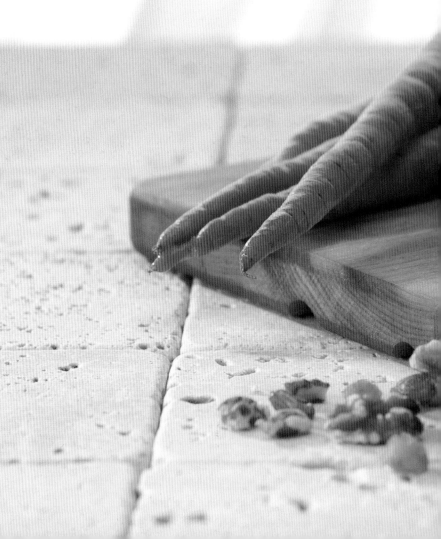

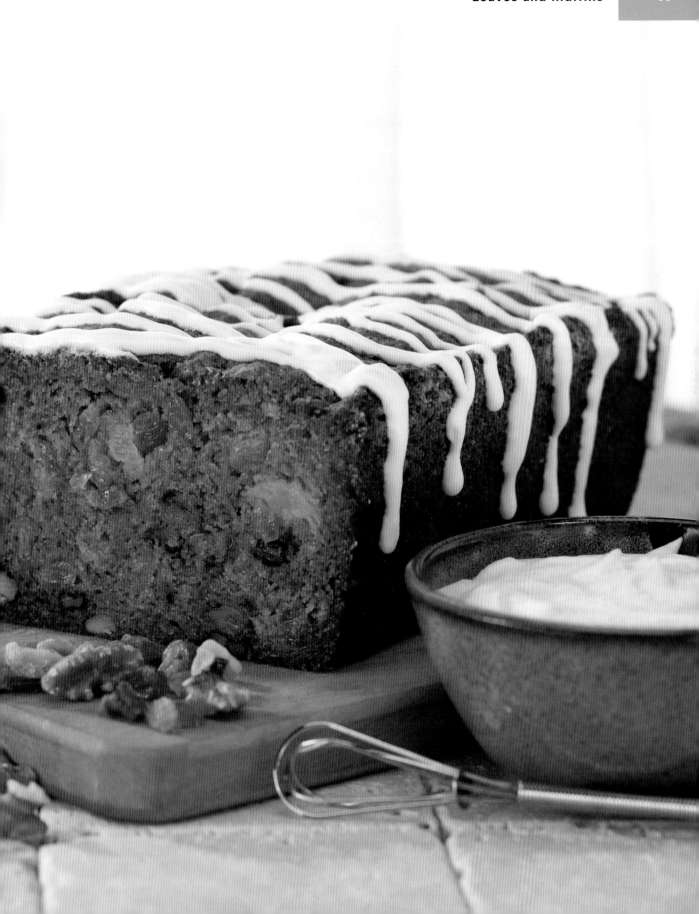

Almond Honey Loaf

Makes 1 loaf

A moist, completely grain- and sucrose-free loaf with just the right amount of sweetness. You can add fruit, carrot or raisins to this loaf. A nutritious snack.

2 ¼ cups (550 mL) finely ground almond meal

¼ cup (60 mL) pea starch

2 tsp (10 mL) xanthan gum

1 tsp (5 mL) baking soda

½ tsp (2 mL) salt

3 large eggs, room temperature (see page 6)

½ cup (125 mL) honey

2 Tbsp (30 mL) egg whites, room temperature

2 Tbsp (30 mL) oil

Preheat oven to 335°F (170°C). Mix first 5 ingredients in an extra-large bowl.

Mix last 4 ingredients in a separate bowl. Fold egg mixture into almond meal mixture until all dry mixture is wet. Don't beat. Pour batter into a greased 8 x 4 inch (20 x 10 cm) baking pan. Bake in preheated oven for 50 to 60 minutes until wooden pick inserted in centre of loaf comes out clean. Place pan on a wire rack to cool.

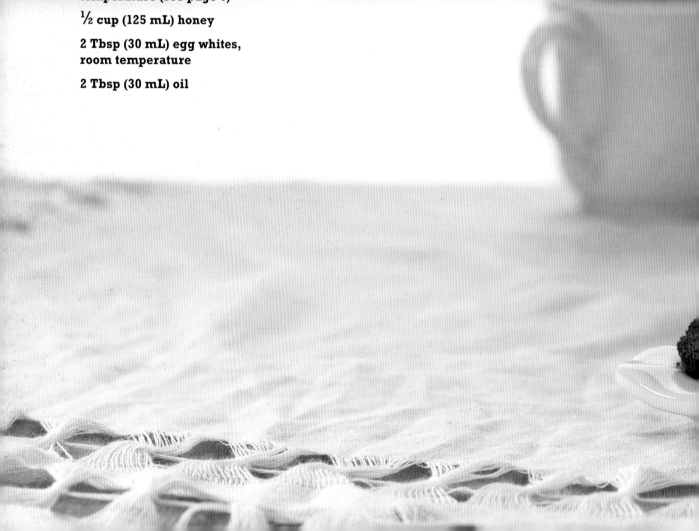

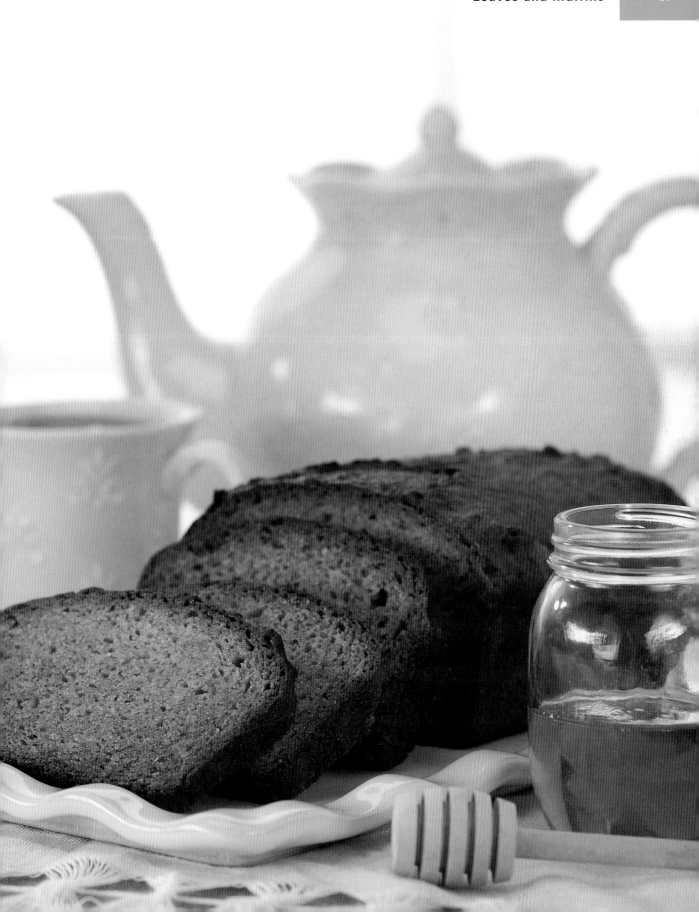

Lemon Cranberry Loaf

Makes 1 loaf

Lemon and cranberry combinations always go well together and this light loaf is no exception. It's part of my regular fall and holiday season fare when fresh cranberries are bountiful.

1 cup (250 mL) sugar

½ cup (125 mL) brown rice flour

½ cup (125 mL) pea starch

½ cup (125 mL) tapioca starch

½ cup (125 mL) white rice flour

2 tsp (10 mL) xanthan gum

1 ½ tsp (7 mL) baking powder

½ tsp (5 mL) salt

½ tsp (2 mL) baking soda

3 large eggs, room temperature (see page 6), beaten

1 cup (250 mL) finely chopped cranberries, fresh or frozen

¼ cup (60 mL) oil

1 tsp (5 mL) orange flavouring

zest from 1 large, fresh organic lemon

¼ to ½ cup (60 to 125 mL) milk

Preheat oven to 350°F (175°C). Mix first 9 ingredients in an extra-large bowl.

Mix next 5 ingredients in a separate bowl. Fold cranberry mixture into flour mixture until all dry mixture is wet. Don't beat. Add milk as needed if batter appears too dry. Pour batter into a greased 8 x 4 inch (20 x 10 cm) baking pan. Bake in preheated oven for 50 to 55 minutes until wooden pick inserted in centre of loaf comes out clean. Place pan on a wire rack to cool.

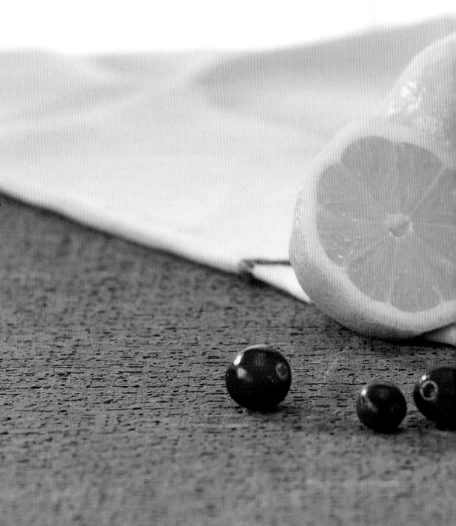

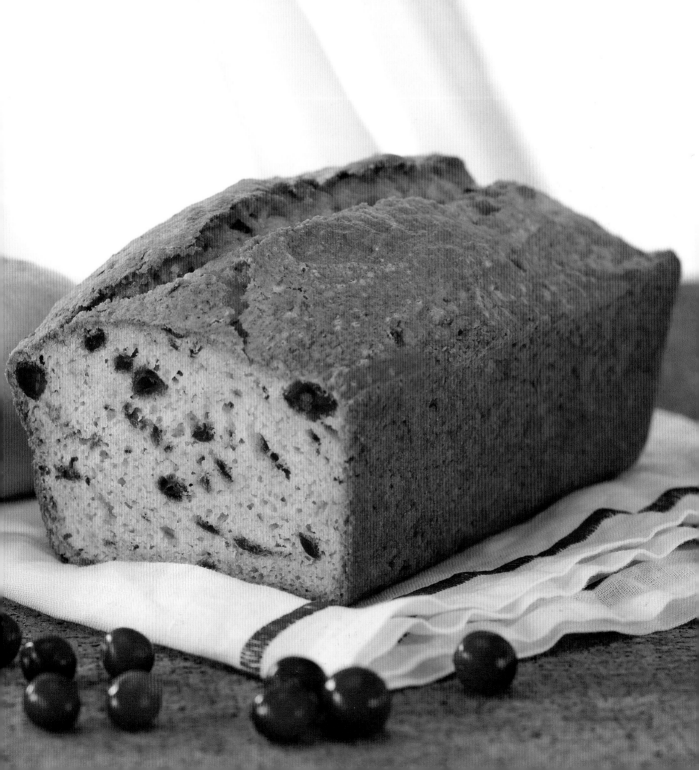

Consumed as a whole food, cranberries have many phytonutrients with numerous health benefits.

Streusel Top Blueberry Muffins

Makes 12

A simple, traditional blueberry muffin with a crunchy streusel topping. Keep any extra streusel in a sealed container in the fridge for your next batch.

¾ cup (175 mL) sugar

½ cup (125 mL) pea starch

½ cup (125 mL) sorghum flour

¼ cup (60 mL) tapioca starch

¼ cup (60 mL) white rice flour

2 tsp (10 mL) baking powder

1 ½ tsp (7 mL) xanthan gum

½ tsp (2 mL) salt

1 ½ cups (375 mL) fresh blueberries (or 1 cup [250 mL] frozen)

¾ cup (175 mL) oil

2 large eggs, room temperature (see page 6)

⅓ to ½ cup (75 to 125 mL) milk

2 Tbsp (30 mL) egg whites, room temperature

1 tsp (5 mL) vanilla

Streusel

½ cup (125 mL) sugar

⅓ cup (75 mL) sweet rice flour

¼ (60 mL) butter, softened

1 tsp (5 mL) cinnamon

Preheat oven to 375°F (190°C). Mix first 8 ingredients in an extra-large bowl.

Blend next 6 ingredients in a separate bowl. Fold blueberry mixture into flour mixture until all dry mixture is wet. Don't beat. Drop batter into a greased 12-count muffin pan with an ice cream scoop (#20 or about ¼ cup [60 mL]).

Combine final 4 ingredients in a separate bowl. Sprinkle over batter. Bake in preheated oven for 30 to 35 minutes until muffins are browned and spring back when lightly pressed. Place pan on a wire rack to cool.

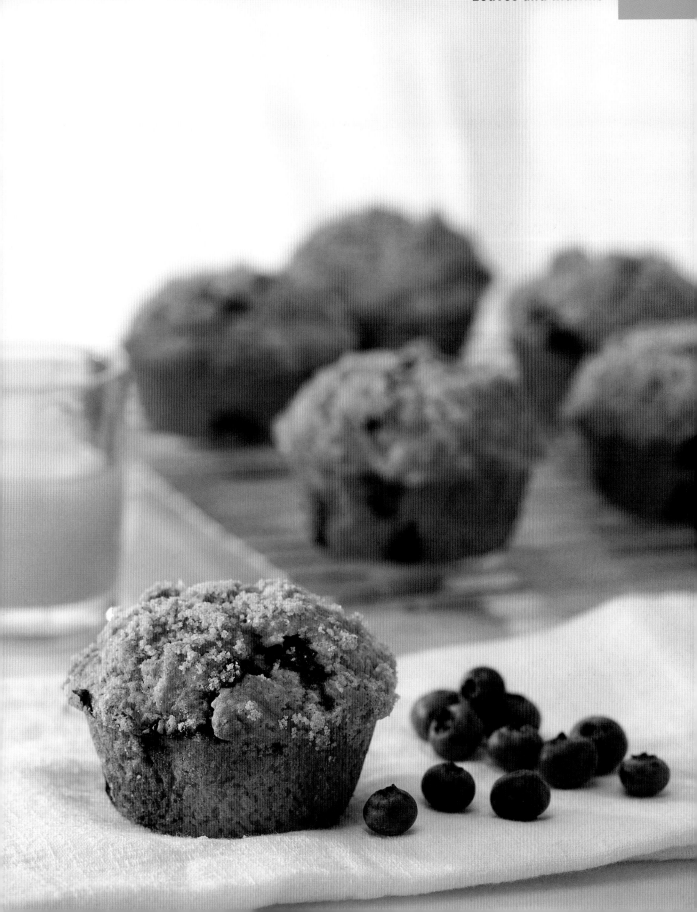

Banana Blueberry Muffins

Makes 12

With the combination of ripe bananas and blueberries, this muffin offers a moist texture with good keeping quality. The flavours of the fruit complement each other and the subtle hint of cinnamon is not overpowering. These muffins freeze well.

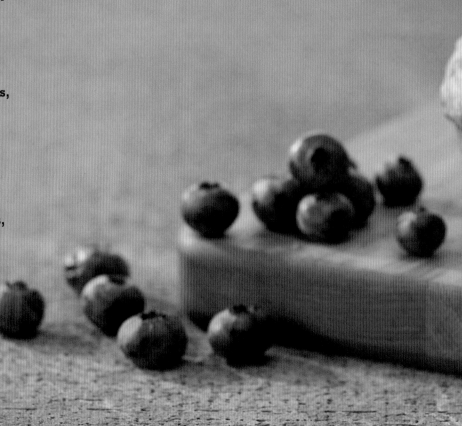

¾ cup (175 mL) sugar

½ cup (125 mL) brown rice flour

½ cup (125 mL) pea starch

½ cup (125 mL) sorghum flour

½ cup (125 mL) tapioca starch

1 Tbsp (15 mL) pea fibre III

1 Tbsp (15 mL) pea fibre 80

2 tsp (10 mL) baking powder

2 tsp (10 mL) xanthan gum

1 tsp (5 mL) cinnamon

½ tsp (2 mL) salt

1 cup (250 mL) blueberries, fresh or frozen

¾ cup (175 mL) oil

3 large eggs, room temperature (see page 6)

2 large ripe bananas

2 Tbsp (30 mL) egg whites, room temperature

1 tsp (5 mL) vanilla

Preheat oven to 400°F (200°C). Mix first 11 ingredients in an extra-large bowl.

Mix last 6 ingredients in a separate bowl. Fold banana mixture into flour mixture until all dry mixture is wet. Don't beat. Drop batter into a greased 12-count muffin pan with an ice cream scoop (#20 or about ¼ cup [60 mL]). Bake in preheated oven for 25 to 30 minutes until muffins are browned and spring back when lightly pressed. Place pan on a wire rack to cool.

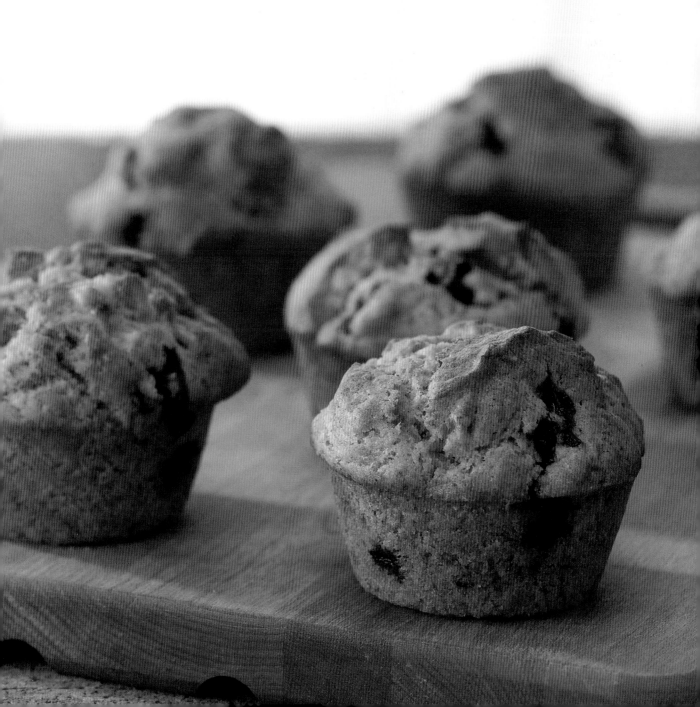

Wild Canadian blueberries are a nutritional powerhouse in a small package. They tend to provide a stronger flavour than cultivated blueberries.

Carrot Muffins

Makes 12

A satisfying, tasty, moist snack for times in between meals. These muffins will last for a day or two, assuming you can keep them from being devoured.

1 cup (250 mL) finely shredded carrot

¾ cup (175 mL) sugar

½ cup (125 mL) brown rice flour

½ cup (125 mL) pea starch

½ cup (125 mL) sorghum flour

½ cup (125 mL) tapioca starch

1 Tbsp (15 mL) pea fibre III

1 Tbsp (15 mL) pea fibre 80

2 tsp (10 mL) baking powder

2 tsp (10 mL) xanthan gum

1 tsp (5 mL) cinnamon

½ tsp (2 mL) salt

⅛ tsp (0.5 mL) ground ginger

¾ cup (175 mL) oil

½ cup (125 mL) crushed pineapple

3 large eggs, room temperature (see page 6)

2 Tbsp (30 mL) egg whites, room temperature

1 tsp (5 mL) vanilla

Preheat oven to 375°F (190°C). Mix first 13 ingredients in an extra-large bowl.

Mix last 5 ingredients in a separate bowl. Fold pineapple mixture into flour mixture until all dry mixture is wet. Don't beat. Drop batter into a greased 12-count muffin pan with an ice cream scoop (#20 or about ¼ cup [60 mL]). Bake in preheated oven for 25 to 30 minutes until muffins are browned and spring back when lightly pressed. Place pan on a wire rack to cool.

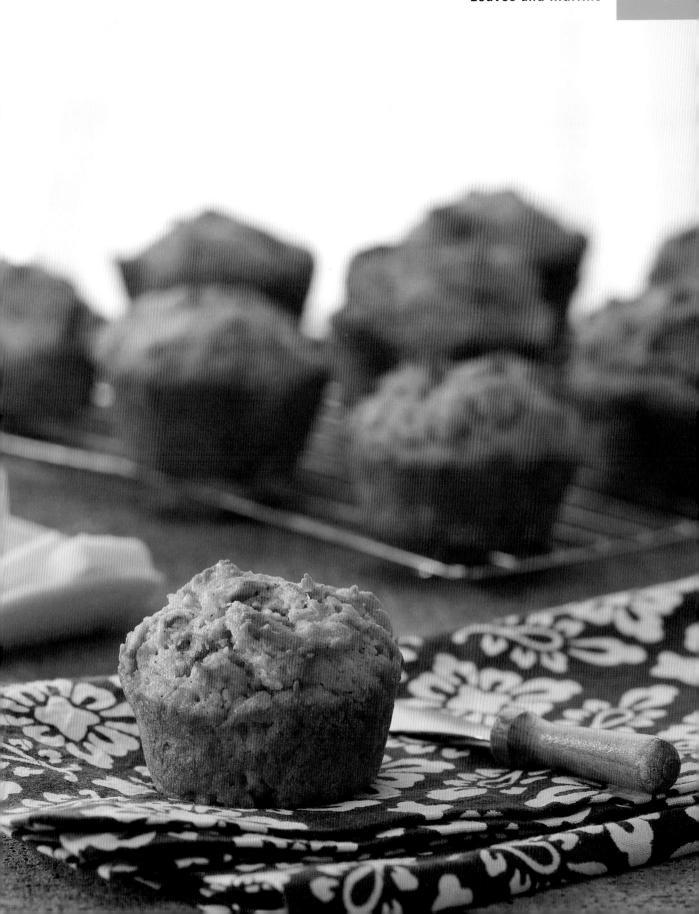

Chocolate Chip Muffins

Makes 12

A classic sweeter muffin loaded with chocolate chips.

1 ½ cups (375 mL) **chocolate chips**

¾ cup (175 mL) **sugar**

½ cup (125 mL) **pea starch**

½ cup (125 mL) **potato starch**

½ cup (125 mL) **tapioca starch**

½ cup (125 mL) **white rice flour**

1 Tbsp (15 mL) **pea fibre 80**

2 tsp (10 mL) **baking powder**

2 tsp (10 mL) **xanthan gum**

1 tsp (5 mL) **cinnamon**

½ tsp (2 mL) **salt**

¾ cup (175 mL) **oil**

3 large **eggs, room temperature (see page 6)**

⅓ cup (75 mL) **water or milk**

2 Tbsp (30 mL) **egg whites, room temperature**

1 tsp (5 mL) **vanilla**

Preheat oven to 375°F (190°C). Mix first 11 ingredients in an extra-large bowl.

Mix last 5 ingredients in a separate bowl. Fold egg mixture into flour mixture until all dry mixture is wet. Don't beat. Drop batter into a greased 12-count muffin pan with an ice cream scoop (#20 or about ¼ cup [60 mL]). Bake in preheated oven for 25 to 30 minutes until muffins are browned and spring back when lightly pressed. Place pan on a wire rack to cool.

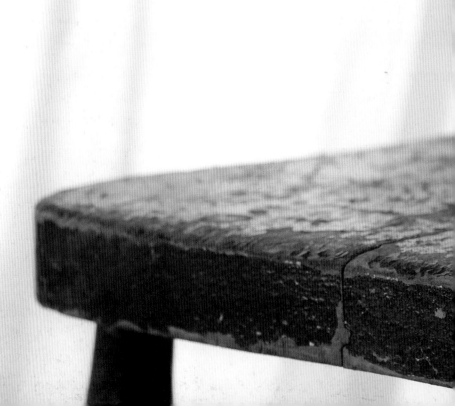

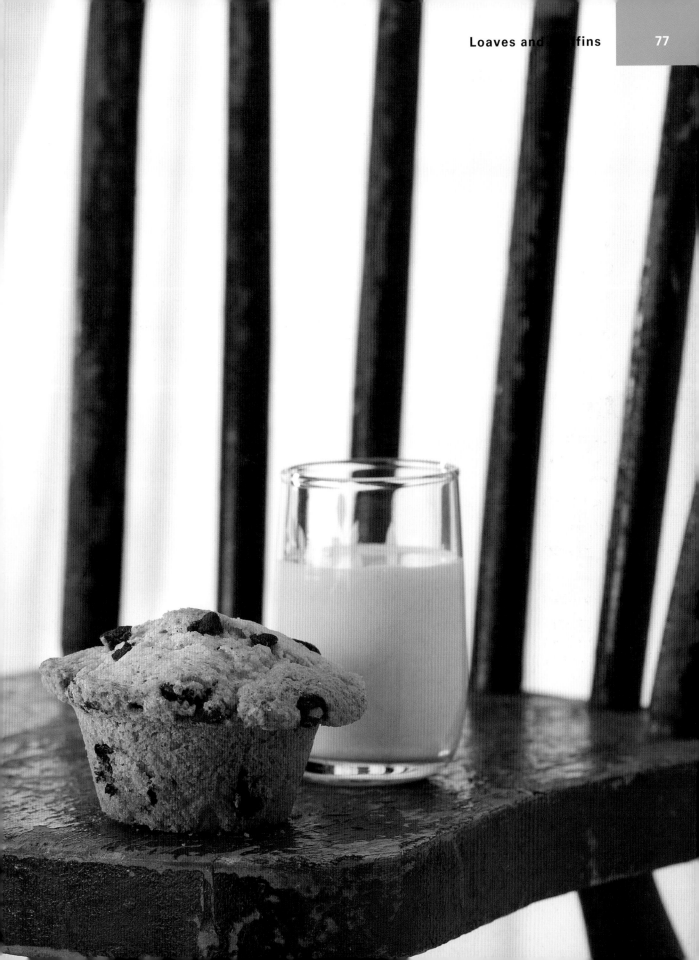

Cranberry Muffins

Makes 12

This muffin is a staple in our house during the fall and holiday season, especially around Thanksgiving and Christmas time. For this recipe, I use dried sweetened cranberries instead of fresh.

1 cup (250 mL) dried sweetened cranberries, cut into pieces

¾ cup (175 mL) sugar

½ cup (125 mL) brown rice flour

½ cup (125 mL) pea starch

½ cup (125 mL) sorghum flour

½ cup (125 mL) tapioca starch

1 Tbsp (15 mL) pea fibre 80

2 tsp (10 mL) baking powder

2 tsp (10 mL) xanthan gum

1 tsp (5 mL) cinnamon

½ tsp (2 mL) salt

¾ cup (175 mL) oil

3 large eggs, room temperature (see page 6)

⅓ cup (75 mL) water or milk

2 Tbsp (30 mL) egg whites, room temperature

1 tsp (5 mL) lemon flavouring

1 tsp (5 mL) vanilla

Preheat oven to 375°F (190°C). Mix first 11 ingredients in an extra-large bowl.

Mix last 6 ingredients in a separate bowl. Fold egg mixture into flour mixture until all dry mixture is wet. Don't beat. Drop batter into a greased 12-count muffin pan with an ice cream scoop (#20 or about ¼ cup [60 mL]). Bake in preheated oven for 25 to 30 minutes until muffins are browned and spring back when lightly pressed. Place pan on a wire rack to cool.

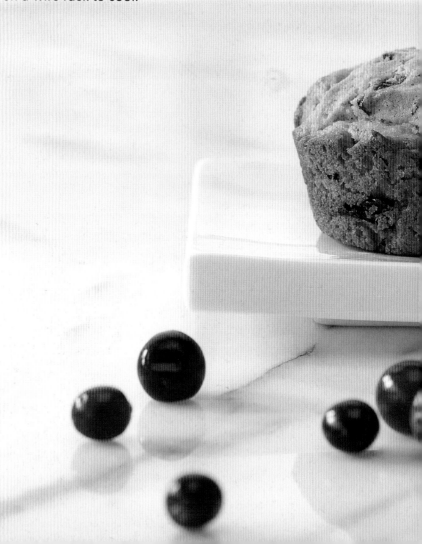

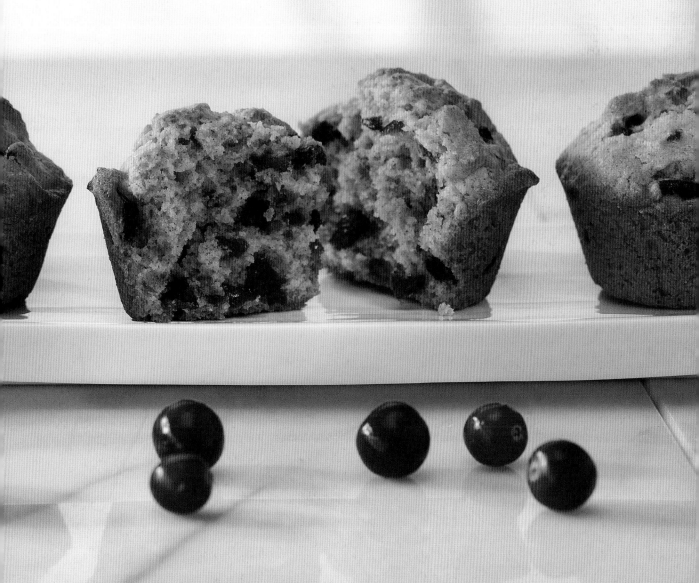

Dried sweetened cranberries can often be used in place of raisins while baking. I also like to use them in trail mixes, or just as a snack on their own.

Chocolate Muffins

Makes 12

Really a mini chocolate cake with the texture of a muffin. Any chocolate lover will enjoy the combination of cocoa and chocolate chips.

1 cup (250 mL) sugar

½ cup (125 mL) cocoa powder

½ cup (125 mL) chocolate chips

½ cup (125 mL) pea starch

½ cup (125 mL) potato starch

½ cup (125 mL) tapioca starch

½ cup (125 mL) white rice flour

1 Tbsp (15 mL) pea fibre III

1 Tbsp (15 mL) pea fibre 80

2 tsp (10 mL) baking powder

2 tsp (10 mL) xanthan gum

1 tsp (5 mL) cinnamon

½ tsp (2 mL) salt

¾ cup (175 mL) oil

3 large eggs, room temperature (see page 6)

⅓ cup (75 mL) water or milk

½ cup (125 mL) applesauce

2 Tbsp (30 mL) egg whites, room temperature

1 tsp (5 mL) vanilla

Preheat oven to 375°F (190°C). Mix first 13 ingredients in an extra-large bowl.

Mix last 6 ingredients in a separate bowl. Fold applesauce mixture into flour mixture until all dry mixture is wet. Don't beat. Drop batter into a greased 12-count muffin pan with an ice cream scoop (#20 or about ¼ cup [60 mL]). Bake in preheated oven for 25 to 30 minutes until muffins are browned and spring back when lightly pressed. Place pan on a wire rack to cool.

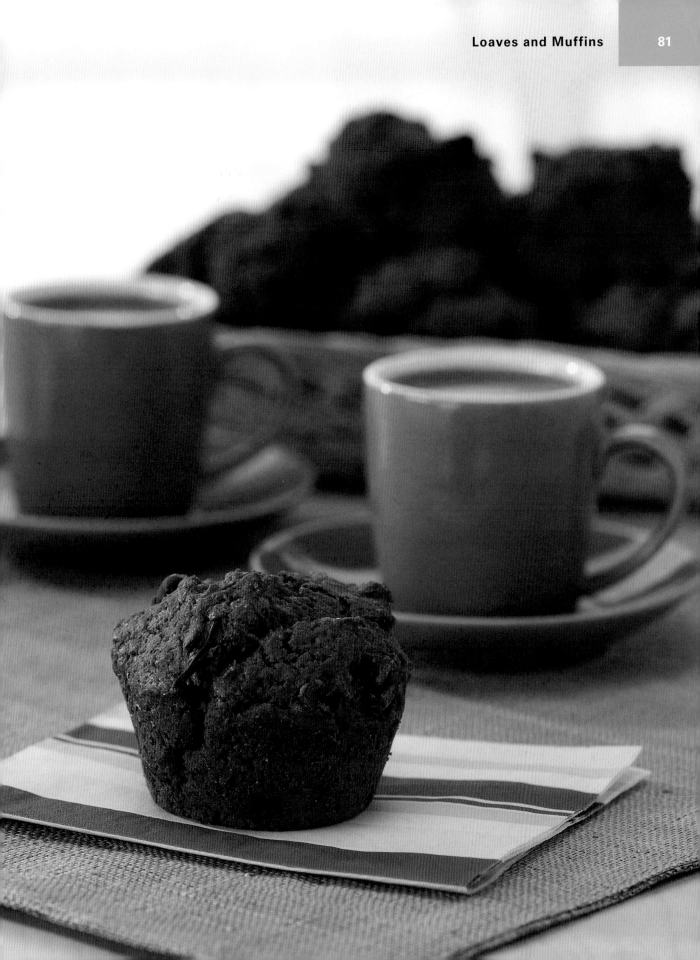

White Cake

Cuts into 12 pieces

A moist, delicate white cake that's not overpowering sweet. Can be enjoyed by itself or with icing and other toppings, such as berries. It's a good base for any birthday cake.

1 cup (250 mL) potato starch

¾ cup (175 mL) sugar

⅓ cup (75 mL) white rice flour

2 Tbsp (30 mL) sweet rice flour

1 Tbsp (15 mL) milk powder

2 tsp (10 mL) baking powder

1 tsp (5 mL) salt

½ tsp (2 mL) baking soda

½ tsp (2 mL) xanthan gum

4 large eggs, room temperature (see page 6)

¾ cup (175 mL) oil

¾ cup (175 mL) water

1 tsp (5 mL) vanilla

Preheat oven to 350°F (175°C). Mix first 9 ingredients in a large bowl.

Blend last 4 ingredients in an extra-large bowl. Fold flour mixture into egg mixture until all dry mixture is wet. Don't overmix. Pour batter into a greased 9 to 10 inch (23 to 25 cm) round or square baking pan. Bake in preheated oven for 50 minutes until wooden pick inserted in centre of cake comes out clean. Place pan on a wire rack to cool.

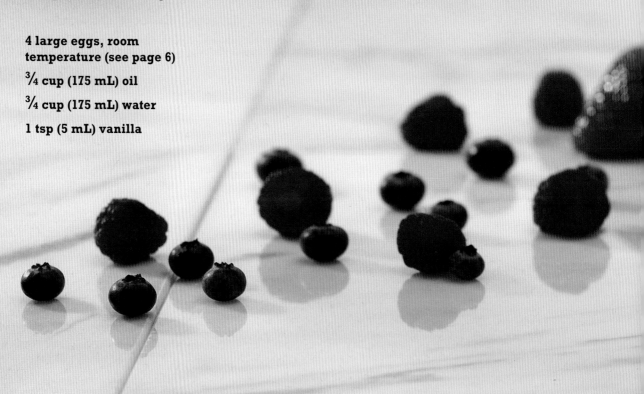

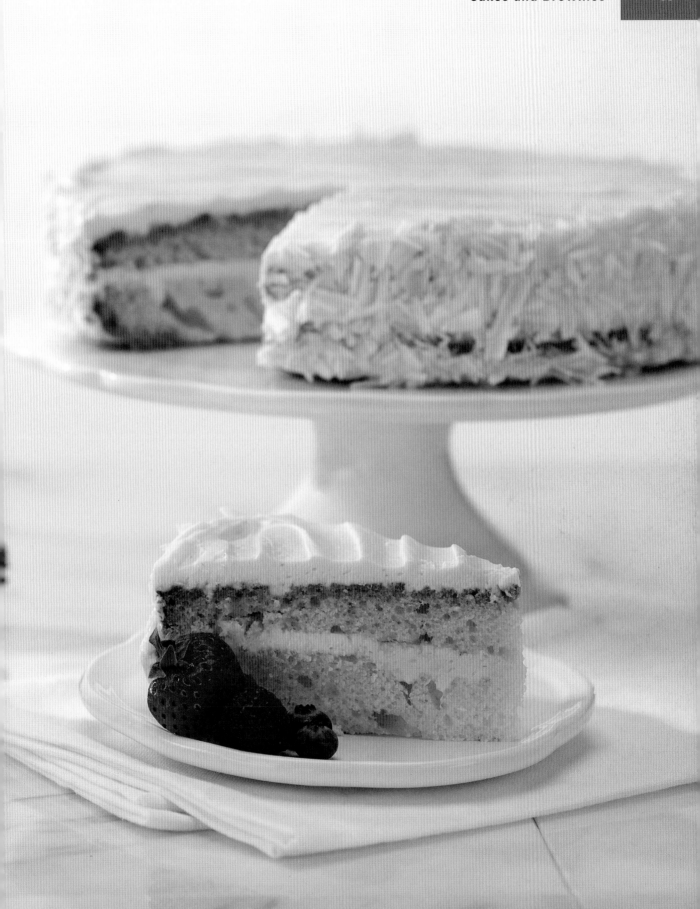

Chocolate Cake

Cuts into 12 pieces

A perfect chocolate cake that's rich in taste, easy to make and soft for days. Enjoy it plain or with your favourite icing, garnished with chocolate curls.

1 cup (250 mL) potato starch

1 cup (250 mL) sugar

½ cup (125 mL) cocoa powder

⅓ cup (75 mL) white rice flour

2 Tbsp (30 mL) sweet rice flour

1 Tbsp (15 mL) milk powder

1 ½ tsp (7 mL) baking powder

1 tsp (5 mL) salt

½ tsp (2 mL) baking soda

½ tsp (2 mL) xanthan gum

4 large eggs, room temperature (see page 6)

¾ cup (175 mL) oil

¾ cup (175 mL) water

1 tsp (5 mL) vanilla

Preheat oven to 350°F (175°C). Mix first 10 ingredients in a large bowl.

Blend last 4 ingredients in an extra-large bowl. Fold flour mixture into egg mixture until all dry mixture is wet. Don't overmix. Pour batter into a greased 9 to 10 inch (23 to 25 cm) round or square baking pan. Bake in preheated oven for 50 minutes until wooden pick inserted in centre of cake comes out clean. Remove from oven and place on a wire rack to cool.

A friend of mine told me she uses tomato juice or tomato soup in place of water when baking, with excellent results.

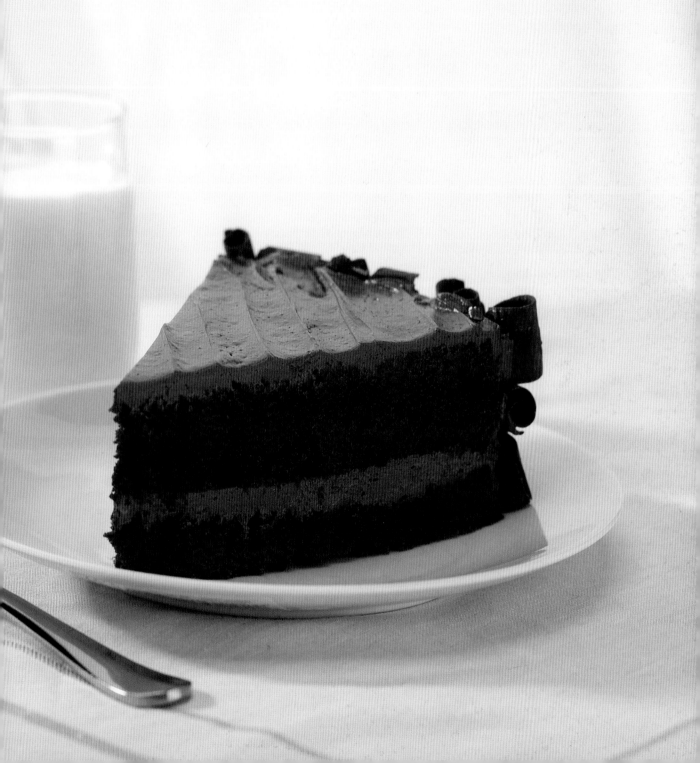

Poppy Seed Coffee Cake

Cuts into 12 wedges

Another favourite coffee cake of mine. The lemon and poppy seed combination is a winner at every typical European table.

1 cup (250 mL) potato starch

¾ cup (175 mL) sugar

½ cup (125 mL) poppy seeds

⅓ cup (75 mL) white rice flour

2 Tbsp (30 mL) sweet rice flour

1 Tbsp (15 mL) milk powder

2 tsp (10 mL) baking powder

1 ½ tsp (7 mL) baking soda

1 tsp (5 mL) salt

½ tsp (2 mL) xanthan gum

4 large eggs, room temperature (see page 6)

¾ cup (175 mL) oil

¾ cup (175 mL) water

1 tsp (5 mL) lemon flavouring

1 tsp (5 mL) vanilla

Icing (optional)

1 cup (250 mL) icing sugar

1 Tbsp (15 mL) butter

2 Tbsp (30 mL) lemon juice (approximately)

Preheat oven to 350°F (175°C). Mix first 10 ingredients in a large bowl.

Blend last 5 ingredients in an extra-large bowl. Fold flour mixture into egg mixture until all dry mixture is wet. Don't overmix. Pour batter into a greased 9 inch (23 cm) Bundt pan. Bake in preheated oven for 50 minutes until wooden pick inserted in centre of cake comes out clean. Place pan on a wire rack to cool.

If a glaze is desired, mix icing sugar and butter in a small bowl. Add lemon juice as needed until mixture is a pouring consistency. Pour over cake while still slightly warm.

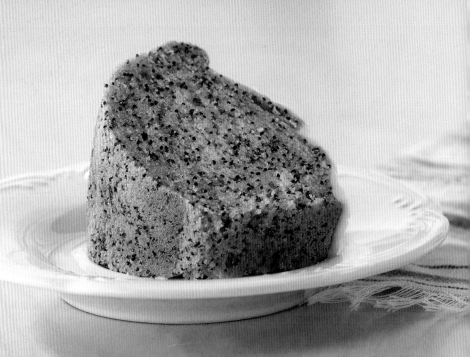

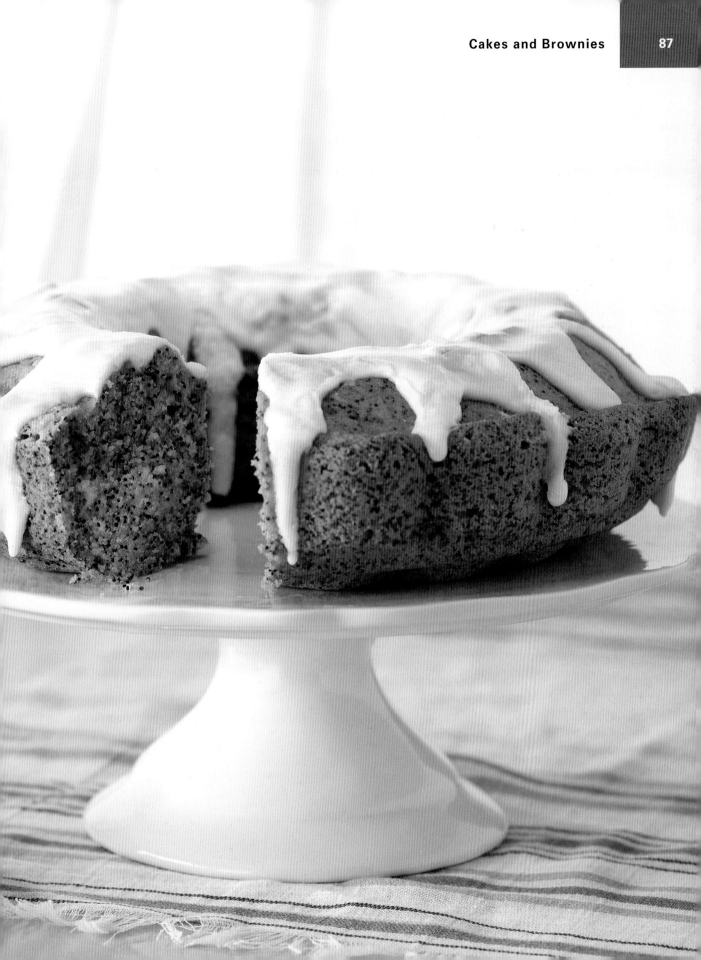

Lemon Cake

Cuts into 12 pieces

Every bite of this moist lemony cake is fresh and refreshing. The lemon sugar glaze supports the full-bodied taste but doesn't overpower the nuances of the lemon peel and lemon flavouring.

1 cup (250 mL) potato starch

¾ cup (175 mL) sugar

⅓ cup (75 mL) white rice flour

2 Tbsp (30 mL) sweet rice flour

1 Tbsp (15 mL) milk powder

1 ½ tsp (7 mL) baking powder

1 tsp (5 mL) salt

1 tsp (5 mL) xanthan gum

½ tsp (2 mL) baking soda

4 large eggs, room temperature (see page 6)

¾ cup (175 mL) oil

¾ cup (175 mL) water

1 tsp (5 mL) lemon flavouring

1 tsp (5 mL) vanilla

grated peel of 1 medium lemon

Glaze

¾ cup (175 mL) icing sugar

1 Tbsp (15 mL) lemon juice

Preheat oven to 350°F (175°C). Mix first 9 ingredients in a large bowl.

Blend next 6 ingredients in an extra-large bowl. Fold flour mixture into egg mixture until all dry mixture is wet. Don't overmix. Pour batter into a greased 9 to 10 inch (23 to 25 cm) round or square baking pan. Bake in preheated oven for 50 minutes until wooden pick inserted in centre of cake comes out clean. Place on a wire rack to cool.

Mix icing sugar and lemon juice in a small bowl. Pour glaze over cake while still slightly warm.

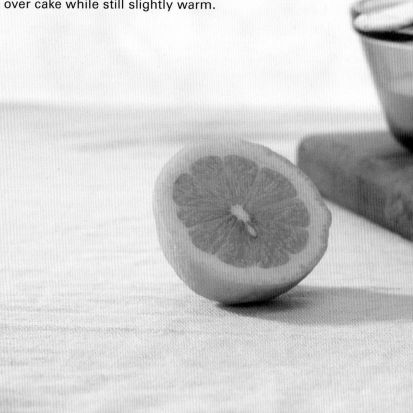

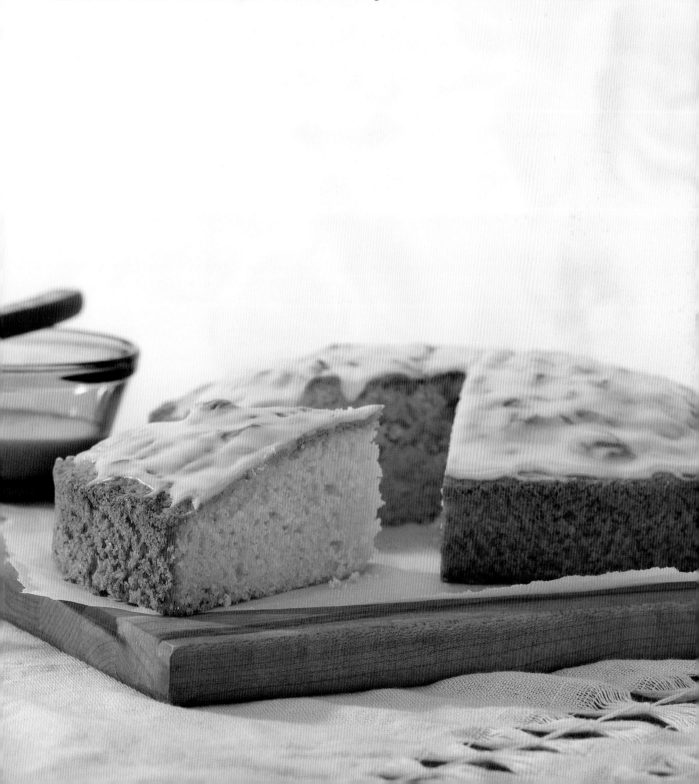

In Germany, we used to call a similar cake Blitzkuchen, which freely translated means "lightning cake," because it was so fast to bake. We sometimes used a flat baking sheet.

Apple Streusel Cake

Cuts into 12 wedges

Apples, raisins and streusel make up the power trio for this delicious, flavourful cake. Another yearly fall staple in my house, when we use our own apples from our backyard apple tree. This cake, however, does not need to wait—enjoy at any time of the year.

¾ cup (175 mL) potato starch

¾ cup (175 mL) sugar

⅓ cup (75 mL) white rice flour

2 Tbsp (30 mL) milk powder

2 Tbsp (30 mL) sweet rice flour

1 ½ tsp (7 mL) baking powder

1 tsp (5 mL) salt

1 tsp (5 mL) xanthan gum

4 large eggs, room temperature (see page 6)

⅔ cup (150 mL) oil

1 tsp (5 mL) vanilla

3 medium apples, cubed into small pieces

½ cup (125 mL) raisins

2 Tbsp (30 mL) berry sugar

¼ tsp (1 mL) cinnamon

Streusel

½ cup (125 mL) sugar

⅓ cup (75 mL) butter, softened

¼ cup (60 mL) sweet rice flour

1 tsp (5 mL) cinnamon

Preheat oven to 350°F (175°C). Mix first 8 ingredients in an extra-large bowl.

Blend next 3 ingredients in a separate bowl. Fold egg mixture into flour mixture until all dry mixture is wet. Don't overmix. Pour batter into a greased 9 to 10 inch (23 to 25 cm) round springform pan.

Mix next 4 ingredients in a separate bowl. Top batter with apple mixture.

Mix last 4 ingredients in a separate bowl. Spread over apple mixture. Bake in preheated oven for 50 minutes until wooden pick inserted in centre of cake comes out clean. Let stand in pan for 10 minutes. Remove ring and place cake on a wire rack to cool.

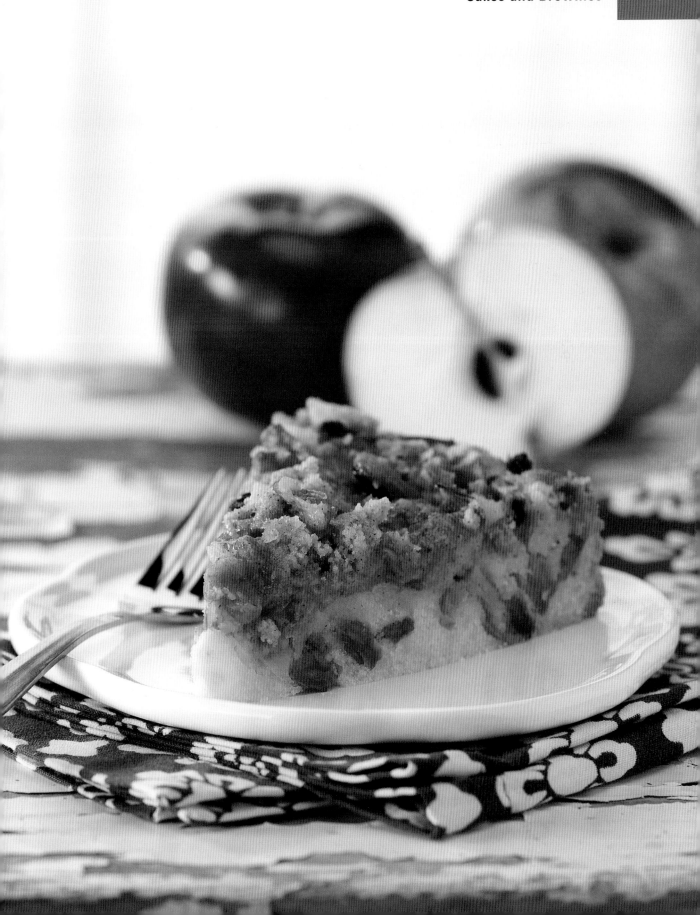

Black Forest Cake

Cuts into 12 wedges

This is it. The one cake that is more like a torte, celebrating the tantalizing combination of chocolate, cherries, cream and Kirsch. Bring this to any function and you will have friends for life. Use real Kirsch, not the imitation kind. Use real whipping cream, not substitutes or cans. This torte will keep in the fridge, but I doubt there will be any leftovers to keep.

1 cup (250 mL) potato starch

1 cup (250 mL) sugar

1/2 cup (125 mL) cocoa powder

1/3 cup (75 mL) white rice flour

2 Tbsp (30 mL) sweet rice flour

1 Tbsp (15 mL) milk powder

1 1/2 tsp (7 mL) baking powder

1 tsp (5 mL) salt

1/2 tsp (2 mL) baking soda

1/2 tsp (2 mL) xanthan gum

4 large eggs, room temperature (see page 6)

3/4 cup (175 mL) oil

3/4 cup (175 mL) water

1 tsp (5 mL) vanilla

2 cups (500 mL) whipping cream

sugar to taste

1/2 cup (125 mL) chocolate

2 Tbsp (30 mL) sugar

1 1/2 tsp (7 mL) Kirsch

2 cups (500 mL) maraschino cherries, plus more for garnish

Preheat oven to 350°F (175°C). Mix first 10 ingredients in a large bowl.

Blend next 4 ingredients in an extra-large bowl. Fold flour mixture into egg mixture until all dry mixture is wet. Don't overmix. Pour batter into a greased 9 to 10 inch (23 to 25 cm) round baking pan. Bake in preheated oven for 50 minutes until wooden pick inserted in centre of cake comes out clean. Place cake upside down on a wire rack to cool.

Whip cream until stiff peaks form. Add sugar to taste and whip. Set aside.

Coarsely grate chocolate. Set aside.

Mix sugar and Kirsch in small bowl. When cake is completely cooled, slice horizontally in half. Lift off top— this is the first half. (The first half of the cake will go on the bottom and the second half will go on the top, because it will be flatter). With a fork, prick top of first half of cake lightly. Drip Kirsch mixture evenly over pricked surface. Spread a thin layer of whipped cream over surface.

Cover evenly with cherries. Top with another layer of whipped cream. Place second half of cake on top. Spread remaining whipped cream all around cake and smooth. Sprinkle grated chocolate over whipped cream. Add cherries on top for decoration.

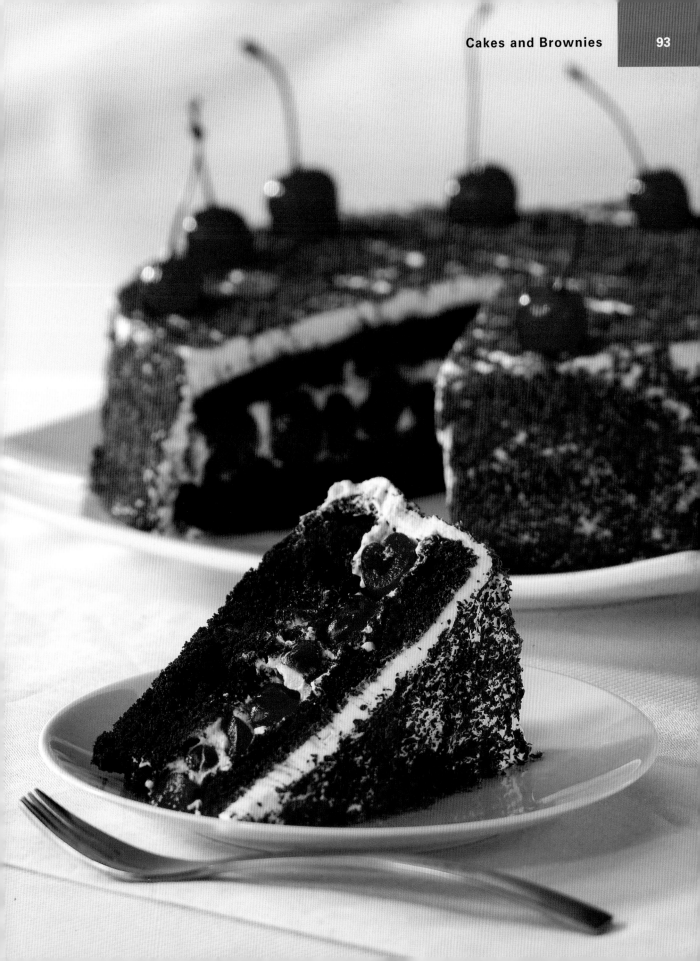

Carrot Cake

Cuts into 12 pieces

Spiced just right, this traditional carrot cake is a mouthwatering delight that will have you coming back for more. It stands well all by itself, but can also be complemented by the traditional cream cheese frosting on page 95 and sprinkled with cinnamon if desired. This cake freezes well.

1 cup (250 mL) potato starch

¾ cup (175 mL) sugar

⅓ cup (75 mL) white rice flour

2 Tbsp (30 mL) sweet rice flour

1 Tbsp (15 mL) milk powder

2 tsp (10 mL) baking powder

1 tsp (5 mL) cinnamon

1 tsp (5 mL) salt

1 tsp (5 mL) xanthan gum

½ tsp (2 mL) baking soda

½ tsp (2 mL) ground ginger

4 large eggs, room temperature (see page 6)

¾ cup (175 mL) oil

¾ cup (175 mL) water

1 tsp (5 mL) vanilla

3 cups (750 mL) grated carrot

½ cup (125 mL) crushed pineapple

Preheat oven to 350°F (175°C). Mix first 11 ingredients in a large bowl.

Blend next 4 ingredients in an extra-large bowl.

Mix carrot and pineapple in a separate bowl. Fold flour mixture and carrot mixture into egg mixture until all dry mixture is wet. Don't overmix. Pour batter into a greased 9 to 10 inch (23 to 25 cm) round or square baking pan. Bake in preheated oven for 50 minutes until wooden pick inserted in centre of cake comes out clean. Place pan on a wire rack to cool. Ice with cream cheese frosting on page 95.

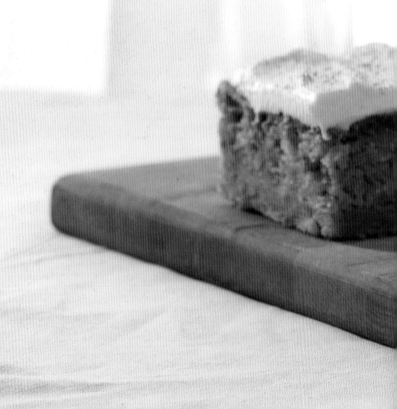

Cream Cheese Frosting

1 cup (250 mL) cream cheese

$\frac{2}{3}$ cup (150 mL) butter

$\frac{1}{4}$ cup (60 mL) honey

1 tsp (5 mL) vanilla

2 $\frac{1}{2}$ to 3 Tbsp (37 to 45 mL) cream

Combine first 4 ingredients in a mixer and beat until fluffy.
Add cream to reach desired spreading consistency.

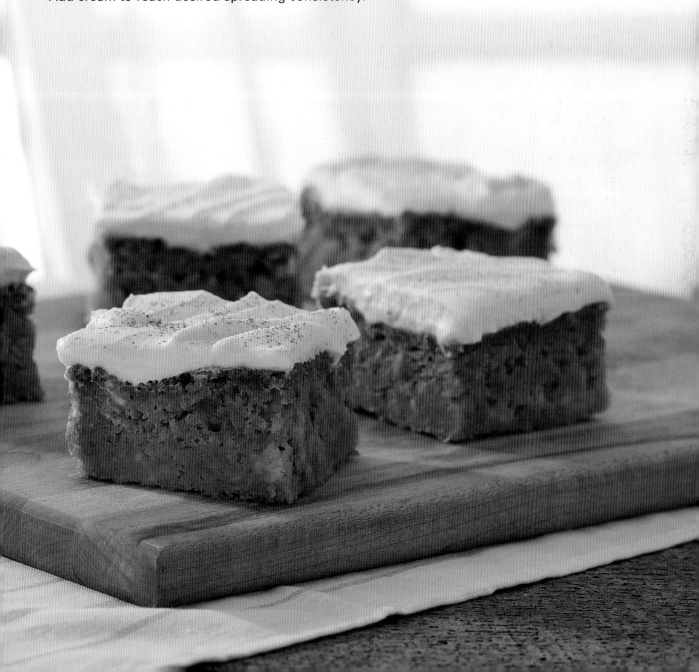

Butterscotch Brownies

Cuts into 12 pieces

A fudgy caramel-flavoured twist on traditional chocolate fudge brownies. These sweet squares are a good addition to any party platter.

½ cup (125 mL) pea starch

½ cup (125 mL) soya flour

½ cup (125 mL) white rice flour

1 Tbsp (15 mL) pea fibre 80

2 tsp (10 mL) baking powder

½ tsp (2 mL) salt

½ cup (125 mL) shortening

2 cups (500 mL) brown sugar

3 large eggs, room temperature (see page 6)

1 tsp (5 mL) vanilla

1 cup (250 mL) chopped walnuts

Preheat oven to 350°F (175°C). Mix first 6 ingredients in an extra-large bowl.

In an electric mixer, mix shortening and brown sugar together until well blended. Add eggs 1 at a time, beating well after each addition. Add vanilla and walnuts. Fold flour mixture into egg mixture until all dry mixture is wet. Pour batter into a greased 9 x 9 inch (23 x 23 cm) baking pan. Bake in preheated oven for 25 to 30 minutes until wooden pick inserted in centre of brownies comes out clean. Remove from oven and immediately cool in freezer for 10 minutes.

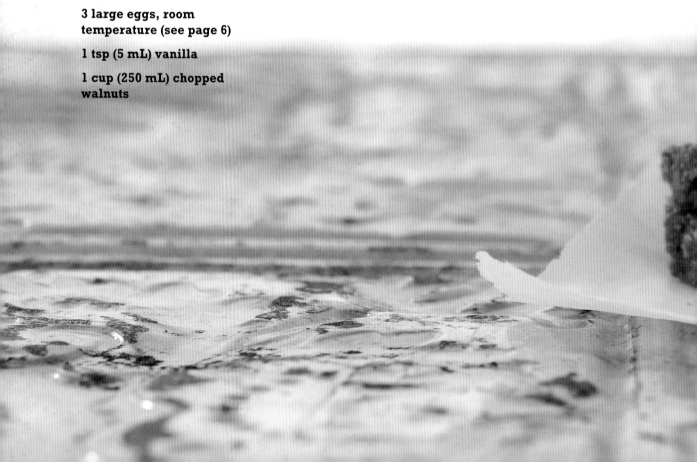

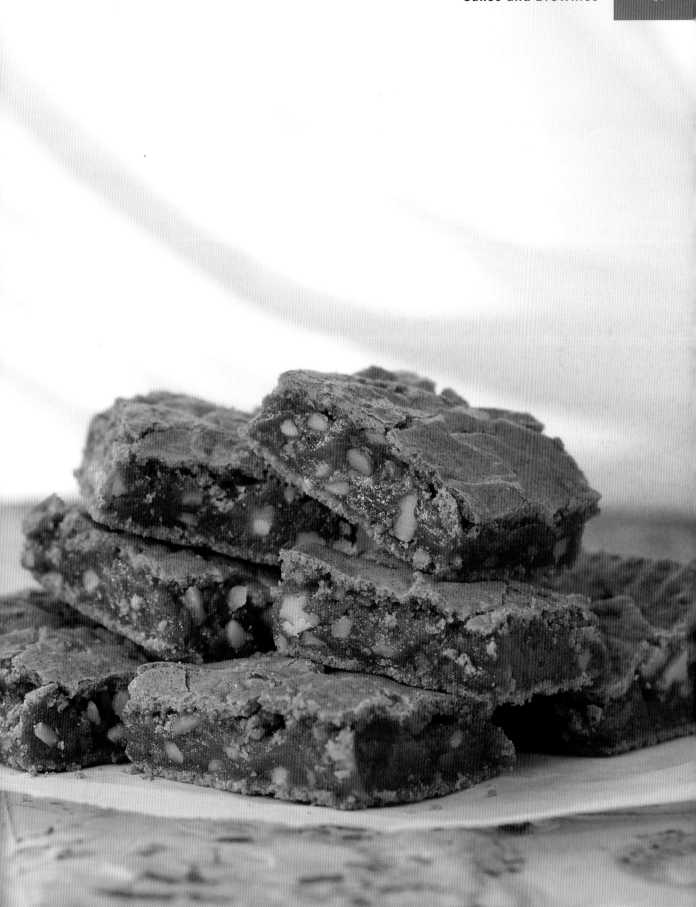

Raisin Coffee Cake

Cuts into 12 wedges

A heavier but still moist pound cake–style dessert that goes well with coffee or tea.

1 cup (250 mL) potato starch

⅓ cup (75 mL) white rice flour

2 Tbsp (30 mL) sweet rice flour

1 Tbsp (15 mL) milk powder

2 tsp (10 mL) baking powder

1 tsp (5 mL) salt

1 tsp (5 mL) xanthan gum

½ tsp (2 mL) baking soda

¼ tsp (1 mL) cinnamon

4 large eggs, room temperature (see page 6)

¾ cup (175 mL) sugar

¾ cup (175 mL) Thompson raisins

¾ cup (175 mL) water

⅔ cup (150 mL) butter

1 tsp (5 mL) vanilla

½ tsp (2 mL) rum flavouring

Glaze

¾ cup (175 mL) icing sugar

1 Tbsp (15 mL) lemon juice

Preheat oven to 350°F (175°C). Mix first 9 ingredients in a large bowl.

Blend next 7 ingredients in an extra-large bowl. Fold flour mixture into egg mixture until all dry mixture is wet. Don't overmix. Pour batter into a greased 9 to 10 inch (23 to 25 cm) Bundt pan. Bake in preheated oven for 50 minutes until wooden pick inserted in centre of cake comes out clean. Remove from oven and place on a wire rack to partially cool.

Mix icing sugar and lemon juice in a small bowl. While cake is still warm, brush with glaze.

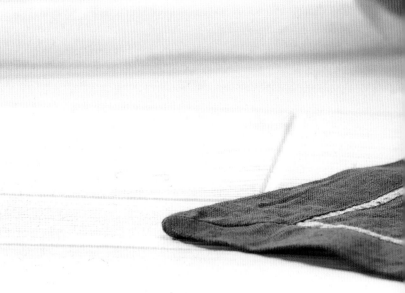

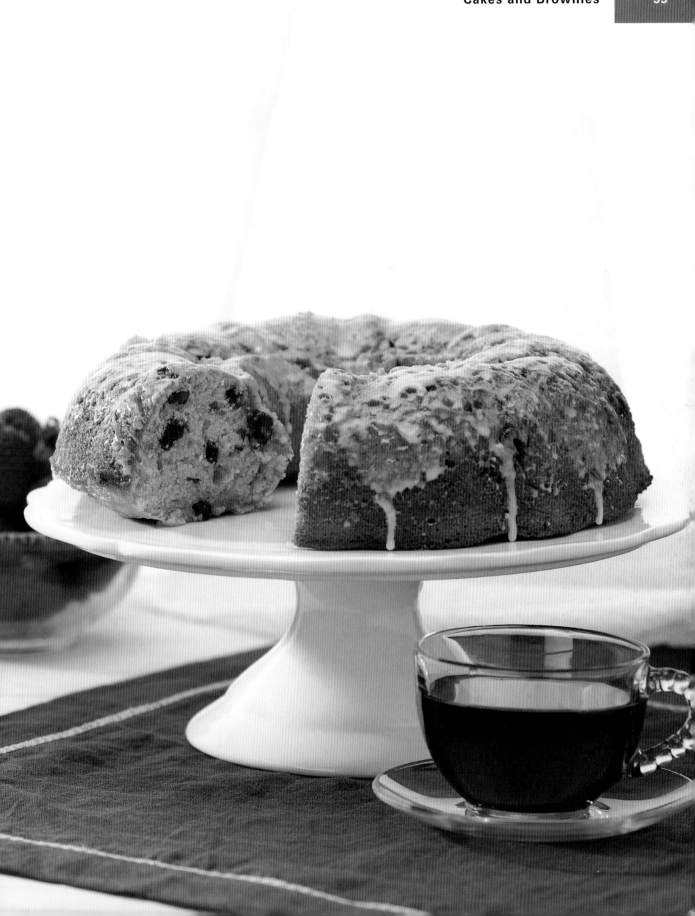

Danish

Makes about 15 large Danishes or about 26 small Danishes

A cake-style Danish that has a traditional appearance with filling and white icing.

1 cup (250 mL) water

2 Tbsp (30 mL) active dry yeast

2 Tbsp (30 mL) sugar

1 cup (250 mL) potato starch

1 cup (250 mL) tapioca starch

1 cup (250 mL) white rice flour

$\frac{2}{3}$ cup (150 mL) sugar

$\frac{1}{4}$ cup (60 mL) whey powder

1 $\frac{1}{2}$ Tbsp (25 mL) pea fibre 80

2 $\frac{1}{2}$ tsp (12 mL) xanthan gum

1 tsp (5 mL) salt

6 Tbsp (90 mL) butter

2 large eggs, room temperature (see page 6)

2 egg yolks, room temperature

2 tsp (10 mL) lemon flavouring

1 tsp (5 mL) vanilla

your favourite jam or Danish filling

Icing

1 cup (250 mL) icing sugar

2 Tbsp (30 mL) water

1 Tbsp (15 mL) butter

Place first 3 ingredients in a small bowl. Set aside.

Mix next 8 ingredients in a large bowl.

Blend next 5 ingredients in an extra-large bowl. Add half of flour mixture to butter mixture and mix. Add yeast mixture to butter mixture and mix. Add rest of flour mixture and mix until batter is smooth.

Spoon 2 to 3 Tbsp (30 to 45 mL) scoops onto parchment paper–lined baking sheet. Spread into rounds with wet spoon and swirl circular depression in each Danish. Fill depressions with 2 Tbsp (30 mL) jam or Danish filling. Let rise for about 20 minutes until doubled in size. Bake in a 350°F (175°C) oven for 20 to 25 minutes until golden. Remove from oven and place on a wire rack to cool.

Combine last 3 ingredients in a small bowl to make a thick white icing. You can adjust icing thickness by adding more icing sugar if needed. Drizzle icing over cooled Danishes.

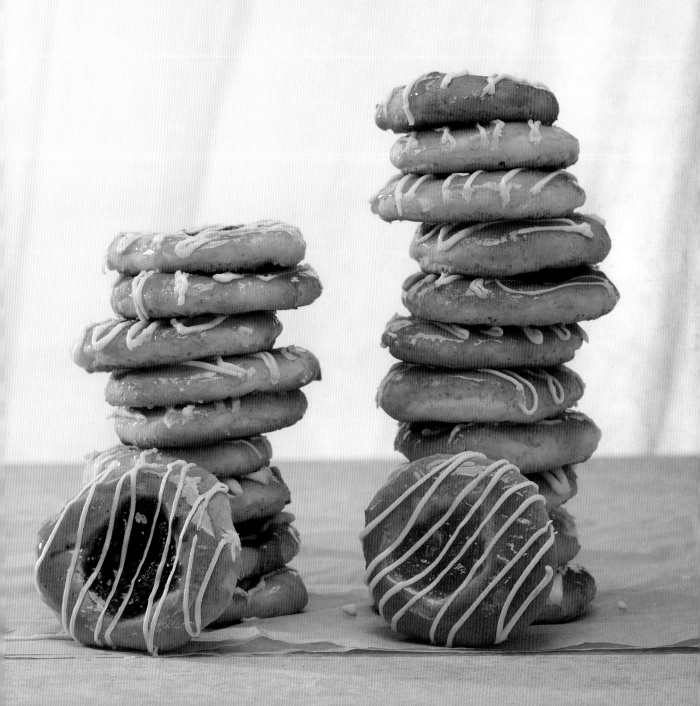

Did you know that the origin of the Danish is attributed to foreign workers coming to Denmark during a bakery strike in 1850?

Light Fruitcake

Makes 1 loaf

This fruit-filled holiday cake is my preferred alternative to the typical, very dark and heavy fruitcakes found in stores. The baking times are long and necessary because of the lower temperatures and high density of the cake. Properly baked, this fruitcake will last for weeks and can be eaten throughout the season, without refrigeration.

1 ½ cups (375 mL) white rice flour

½ cup (125 mL) pea starch

¼ cup (60 mL) soya flour

¼ cup (60 mL) tapioca starch

2 Tbsp (30 mL) pea fibre 80

1 Tbsp (15 mL) baking powder

1 ¼ tsp (6 mL) baking soda

1 ¼ tsp (6 mL) salt

3 cups (750 mL) mincemeat

1 ½ cups (375 mL) sweetened condensed milk

2 large eggs, room temperature (see page 6)

1 cup (250 mL) glazed fruit mix

½ cup (125 mL) glazed green cherries

½ cup (125 mL) glazed red cherries

Preheat oven to 300°F (150°C). Thoroughly mix first 8 ingredients together in a large bowl.

Beat together last 6 ingredients in an extra-large bowl. Add flour mixture to mincemeat mixture. Mix well. The batter might look rather thin. Pour into 8 x 4 inch (20 x 10 cm) baking pan lined with fruitcake paper or double-layered parchment paper. Bake in preheated oven for 2 hours. Reduce heat to 200°F (95°C). Bake for another 45 minutes. Place pan on a wire rack to cool. Let cool completely before slicing.

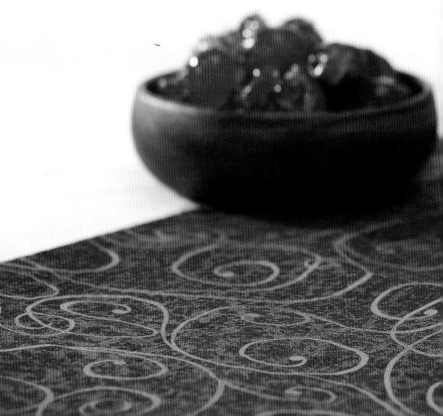

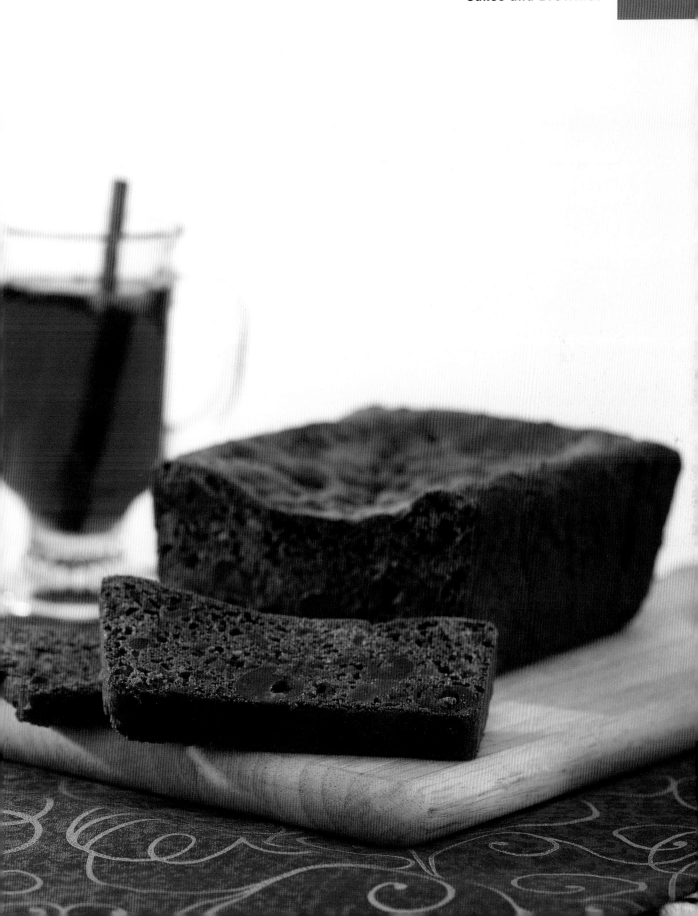

Sponge Cake

Cuts into 12 wedges

A light fluffy cake that can be quickly iced with a sugar icing or used as a base for tortes and fresh fruity cakes. A quick raspberry compote makes a nice topping: just purée 1 cup (250 mL) raspberries, 3 Tbsp (45 mL) honey and 1 Tbsp (15 mL) white wine together until smooth.

1 cup (250 mL) potato starch

⅓ cup (75 mL) tapioca starch

3 Tbsp (45 mL) white rice flour

¾ Tbsp (11 mL) baking powder

¾ tsp (4 mL) salt

½ tsp (2 mL) cream of tartar

6 large eggs, room temperature (see page 6)

1 ⅛ cups (280 mL) sugar

1 ½ tsp (7 mL) vanilla

Preheat oven to 350°F (175°C). Mix first 6 ingredients in a large bowl.

Beat eggs in a separate large bowl for about 10 minutes until fluffy. Add sugar very slowly, beating after each addition. Add vanilla slowly. Fold flour mixture into egg mixture slowly until all dry mixture is wet. Pour batter into a 10 inch (25 cm) round springform pan. Bake for 30 to 40 minutes until cake springs back to the touch. Place pan on a wire rack to cool. Glace with an icing if desired or serve with fruit compote.

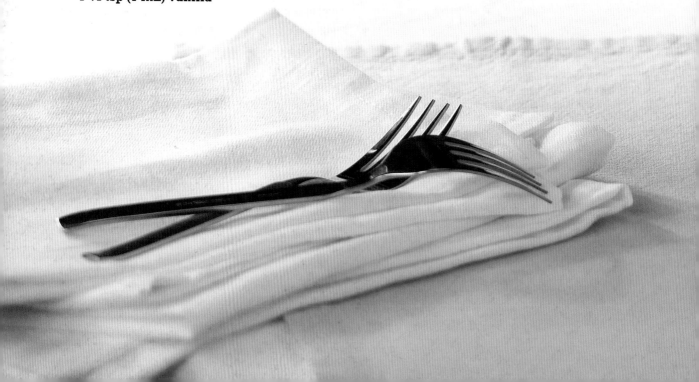

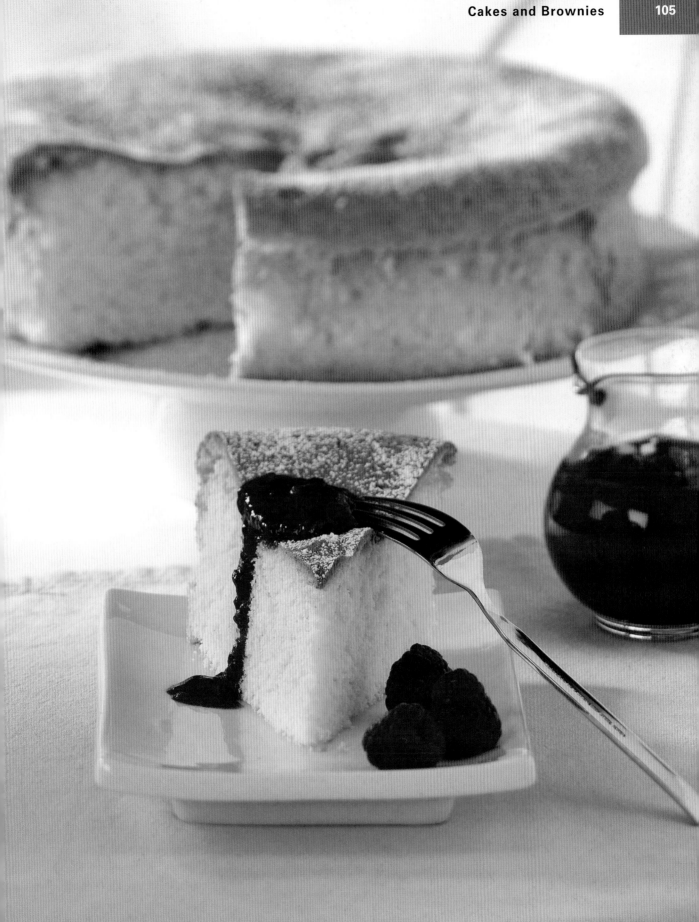

Jelly Roll

Cuts into 12 to 18 slices

Jelly rolls look so pretty when assembled and this cake provides the perfect roll base. So light that it doesn't distract from your choice of filling.

³⁄₄ cup (175 mL) potato starch

¹⁄₄ cup (60 mL) tapioca starch

2 Tbsp (30 mL) white rice flour

³⁄₄ Tbsp (11 mL) baking power

¹⁄₂ tsp (2 mL) cream of tartar

¹⁄₂ tsp (2 mL) salt

6 large eggs, room temperature (see page 6)

1 ¹⁄₈ cups (280 mL) sugar

1 ¹⁄₂ tsp (7 mL) vanilla

Preheat oven to 350°F (175°C). Line a baking sheet with sides with parchment paper, leaving some overhang on sides. Mix first 6 ingredients in a medium bowl.

Beat eggs in an extra-large bowl for about 10 minutes until fluffy. Add sugar very slowly, beating after each addition. Add vanilla slowly. Slowly fold flour mixture into egg mixture until all dry mixture is wet. Pour batter into parchment paper–lined baking sheets. Bake in preheated oven for 12 to 15 minutes. Remove paper and jelly roll cake from baking sheet. Let cool until cake is slightly warm. Place upside down on a clean tea towel. Remove paper carefully. Spread with your favourite jam, filling or butter crème and roll it up. Cut into ¹⁄₂ to 1 inch (12 mm to 2.5 cm) slices.

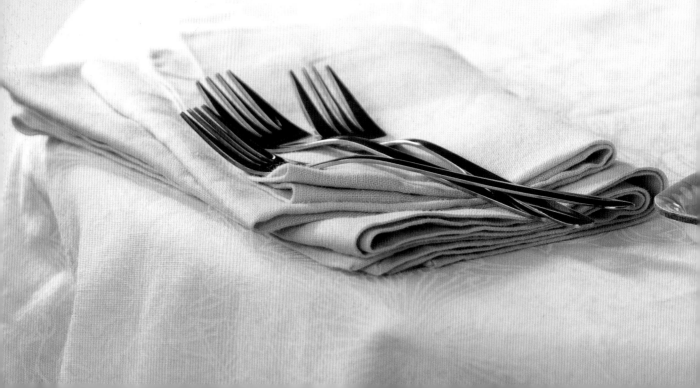

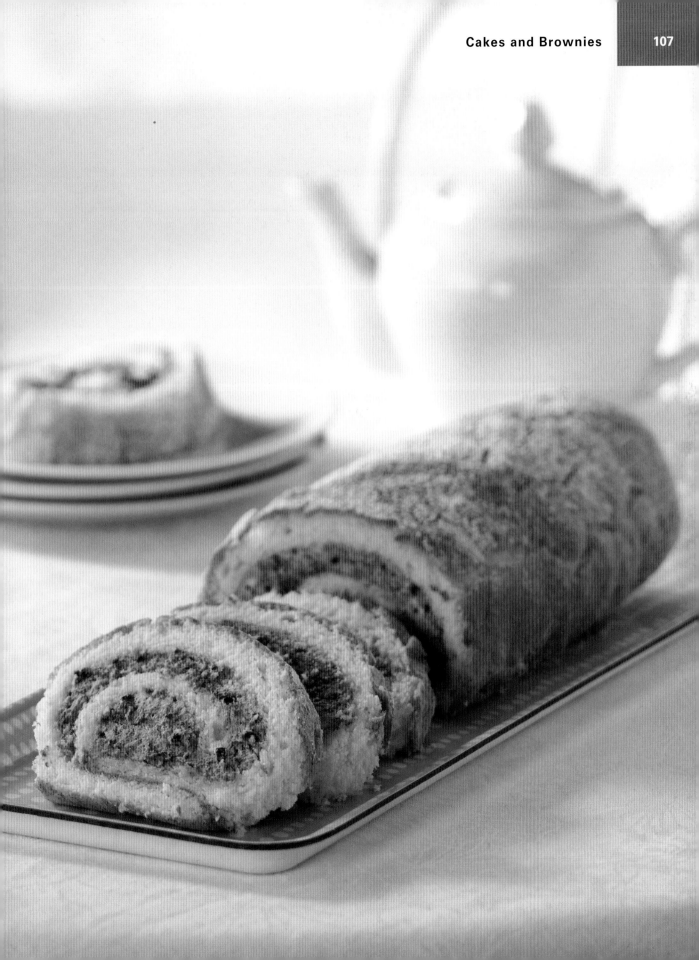

Mocha Butter Crème Cake

Cuts into 12 wedges

You'll have to cut yourself a piece of this delectable cake first at your next coffee date or you might be left without one. A winning combination of chocolate and coffee flavours.

1 cup (250 mL) potato starch

¾ cup (175 mL) sugar

½ cup (125 mL) cocoa powder

⅓ cup (75 mL) white rice flour

¼ cup (60 mL) grated dark chocolate

2 Tbsp (30 mL) sweet rice flour

1 Tbsp (15 mL) instant coffee

1 Tbsp (15 mL) milk powder

1 ½ tsp (7 mL) baking powder

1 tsp (5 mL) salt

1 tsp (5 mL) xanthan gum

½ tsp (2 mL) baking soda

4 large eggs, room temperature (see page 6)

¾ cup (175 mL) oil

¾ cup (175 mL) water

1 tsp (5 mL) vanilla

Butter Crème

½ cup (125 mL) butter

½ cup (125 mL) shortening

1 tsp (5 mL) vanilla

4 cups (1 L) icing sugar

2 Tbsp (30 mL) milk

chocolate sprinkles or coffee beans, for decoration

Preheat oven to 350°F (175°C). Mix first 12 ingredients in a large bowl.

Blend next 4 ingredients in an extra-large bowl. Fold flour mixture into egg mixture until all dry mixture is wet. Don't overmix. Pour batter into a greased pan. Bake in preheated oven for 50 minutes until wooden pick inserted in centre of cake comes out clean. Place pan on a wire rack to cool.

Mix butter and shortening in an electric mixer with a wire whisk. Add vanilla. Slowly add icing sugar 1 cup (250 mL) at a time, beating well after each addition at medium speed. Scrape sides and bottom of bowl with spatula after each addition. Slowly add milk and beat on medium until butter crème is light and fluffy.

Once cake is cooled, slice in half horizontally. Lift off top—this is the first half. (The first half of the cake will go on the bottom and the second half will go on top, because it will be flatter.) Spread butter crème evenly over first half. Cover with second half of cake. Spread sides and top of cake with butter crème. Decorate with chocolate sprinkles or coffee beans.

Dutch-processed cocoa is treated with alkali to create a less acidic cocoa powder. It has a darker, richer colour than other cocoa powders.

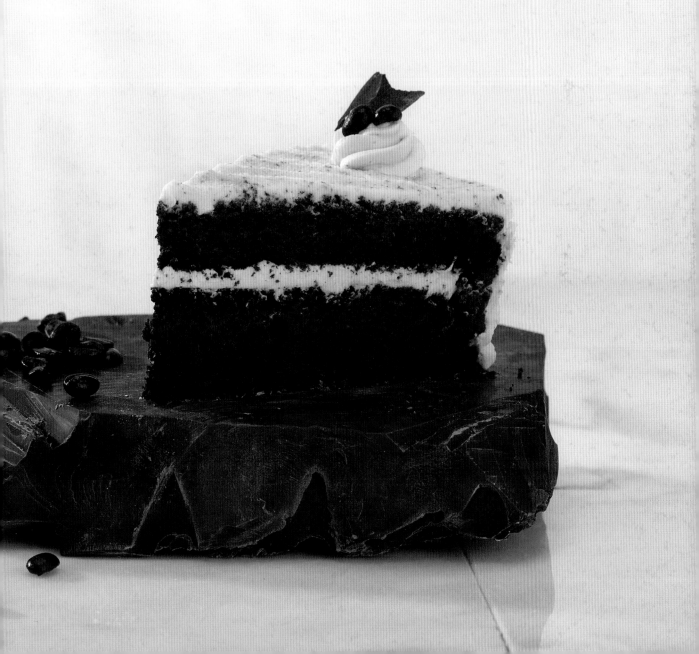

Fruit Sponge Cake

Makes 2; cuts into 24 wedges

The colourful display of fresh fruit in a white fluffy filling on this soft cake is a refreshing hit at any dessert table. I always use the apricot glaze myself.

1 cup (250 mL) potato starch

⅓ cup (75 mL) tapioca starch

3 Tbsp (45 mL) white rice flour

¾ Tbsp (11 mL) baking powder

¾ tsp (4 mL) salt

½ tsp (2 mL) cream of tartar

6 large eggs, room temperature (see page 6)

1 ⅛ cups (280 mL) sugar

1 ½ tsp (7 mL) vanilla

Filling

(double filling recipe if you desire a thicker layer of filling)

1 package (250 mL) cream cheese, softened

½ cup (125 mL) icing sugar, sifted

1 tsp (5 mL) vanilla

½ cup (125 mL) whipping cream

3 cups (750 mL) fruit (such as strawberries or blueberries)

Glaze (optional)

½ cup (125 mL) apricot jam, sieved (discard solids)

1 Tbsp (15 mL) lemon juice

Preheat oven to 350°F (175°C). Mix first 6 ingredients in a medium bowl.

Beat eggs until fluffy in an extra-large bowl. Add sugar very slowly, beating after each addition. Add first amount of vanilla slowly. Slow fold flour mixture into egg mixture until all dry mixture is wet. Divide batter into 2 portions and pour each into a greased or parchment paper–lined 10 to 12 inch (25 to 30 cm) round springform pan. Bake in preheated oven for 35 to 45 minutes until cake springs back to the touch. Remove from oven and place on a wire rack to cool.

Beat next 3 ingredients together until smooth. Whip cream until stiff peaks form. Fold whipped cream into cream cheese mixture. Spread filling over sponge cakes. Cover with fruit of your choice.

If you want to use the glaze, melt apricot jam and lemon juice together. Brush over fruit and serve.

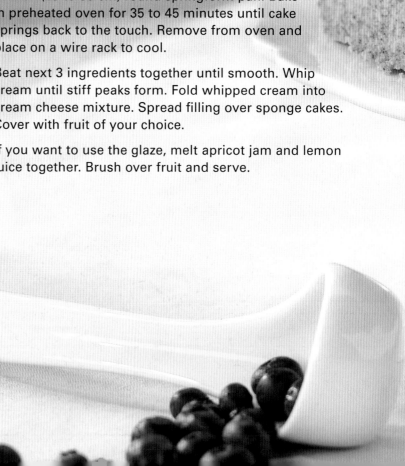

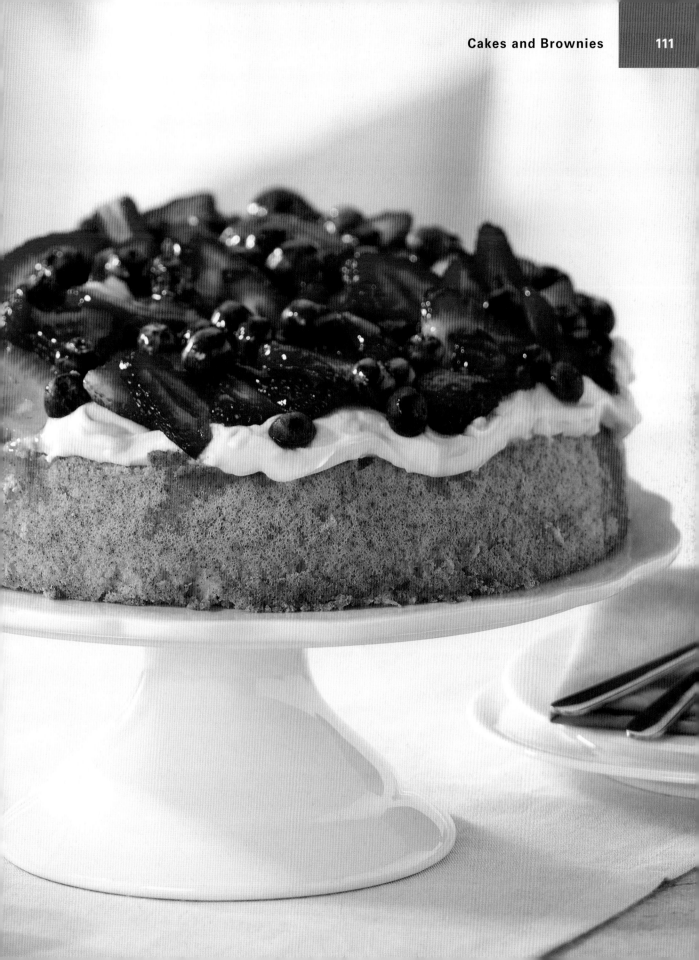

Brownies

Cuts into 12 squares

This brownie recipe offers you a choice of either moist cake-style brownies or a chewier version, depending on how you bake it. I prefer these cake-style brownies to very heavy fudgy-style brownies. The chewy baking method is the perfect compromise between the two and will make everyone happy.

⅓ cup (75 mL) pea starch

⅓ cup (75 mL) potato starch

⅓ cup (75 mL) sweet rice flour

⅓ cup (75 mL) tapioca starch

1 Tbsp (15 mL) pea fibre 80

1 tsp (5 mL) baking powder

1 tsp (5 mL) xanthan gum

½ tsp (2 mL) salt

4 large eggs, room temperature (see page 6)

1 tsp (5 mL) vanilla

2 cups (500 mL) sugar

1 cup (250 mL) butter

1 cup (250 mL) cocoa powder

Preheat oven to 375°F (190°C). Mix first 8 ingredients in an extra-large bowl.

Beat eggs in a separate bowl until fluffy. Add vanilla and sugar slowly, beating well after each addition. Melt butter and add cocoa powder. Slowly add butter mixture to egg mixture. Fold flour mixture into egg mixture until all dry mixture is wet. Pour into a greased 9 x 9 inch (23 x 23 cm) pan. Bake in preheated oven for 30 minutes until wooden pick inserted in centre of brownies comes out clean. Remove from oven and place on a wire rack to cool.

Variation: For chewy brownies, reduce baking time by 3 to 5 minutes. After baking, immediately place brownies in freezer for 10 minutes.

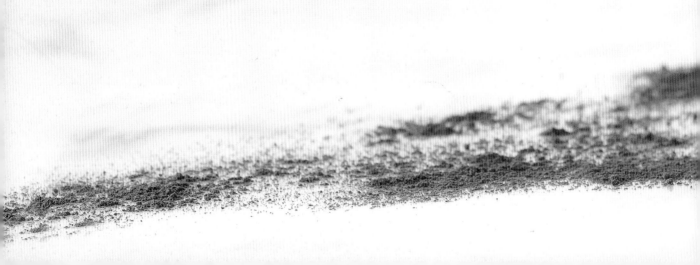

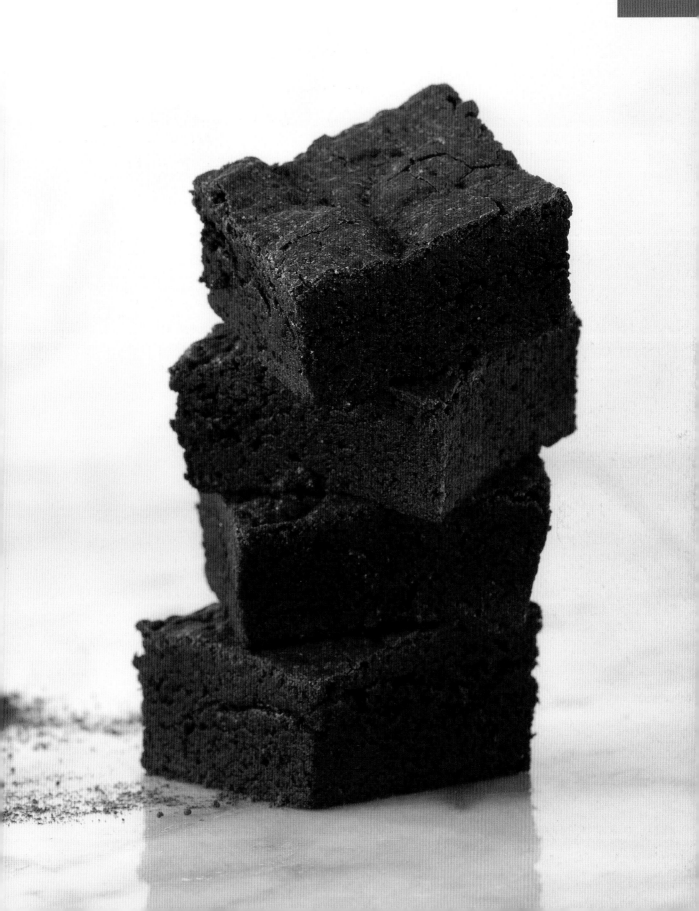

Tender Pie Crust

Makes 1 pie crust (top and bottom)

A nice all-purpose pie crust for any type of filling. You can prebake this crust for cold pie fillings.

1 cup (250 mL) white rice flour

½ cup (125 mL) sweet rice flour

½ cup (125 mL) tapioca starch

1/4 cup (60 mL) pea starch

1 Tbsp (15 mL) pea fibre 80

1 Tbsp (15 mL) sugar

1 ½ tsp (7 mL) xanthan gum

1 tsp (5 mL) baking powder

1 tsp (5 mL) salt

¾ cup (175 mL) shortening or lard

1 large egg, room temperature (see page 6)

2 Tbsp (30 mL) cold water

2 Tbsp (30 mL) vinegar

pie filling

Preheat oven to 450°F (230°C). Mix first 9 ingredients in a large bowl. Cut in shortening or lard.

Lightly beat egg and add to mixture. Add water and vinegar. Dust hands with sweet rice flour. Turn out dough onto surface lightly floured with sweet rice flour. Divide dough into 2 equal balls. Roll each out to about 12 inches (30 cm) or press directly into pie pans.

Fill with your favourite pie filling and bake in preheated oven for 15 minutes. Reduce heat to 350°F (175°C) and bake for another 30 to 35 minutes.

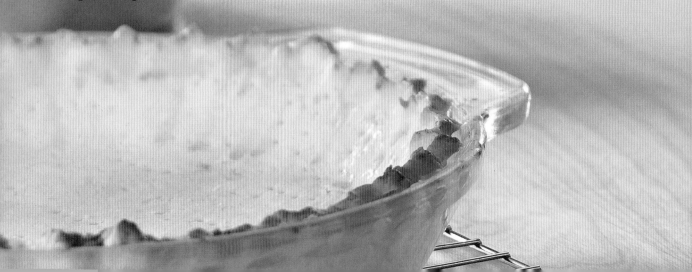

Crumb Crust

Makes 1 pie crust

An easy, no-roll crumb crust for sweet pies or cheesecakes. I like to use crispy cookies such as gingersnaps (see page 128) for this recipe.

Preheat oven to 350°F (175°C). Combine all 4 ingredients in a bowl. Mix together. Press into 9 inch (23 cm) pie pan. Bake in preheated oven for 12 to 15 minutes until crust feels dry to the touch. Use for no-bake fillings or cheesecakes.

2 ½ cups (625 mL) gluten-free graham-style cookies or crackers

⅓ cup (75 mL) shortening

3 Tbsp (45 mL) berry sugar

1 ½ tsp (7 mL) sweet rice flour

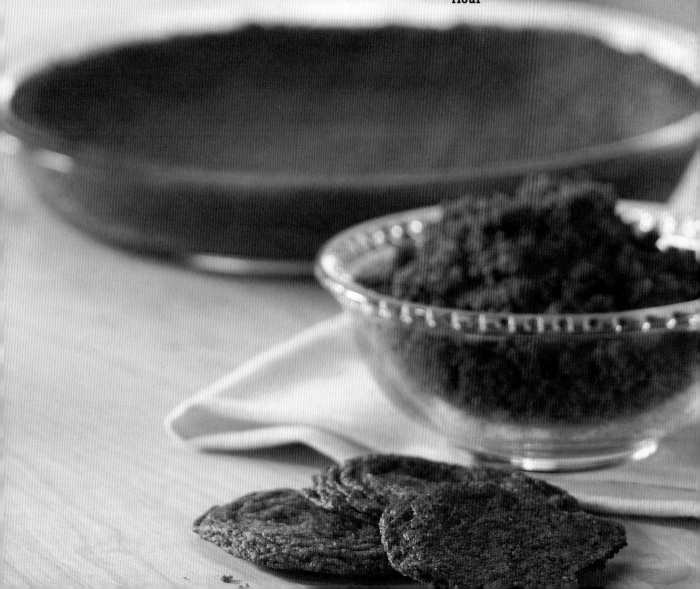

Apple Pie

Cuts into 8 wedges

I can't believe we never really had apple pie in Germany. This recipe makes a delicious apple pie that always calls for at least two slices. I like hardy, tart apples for this recipe. Serve with whipped cream and cinnamon if desired.

4 cups (1 L) thinly sliced apples

1 Tbsp (15 mL) lemon juice

¾ cup (175 mL) water

¼ cup (60 mL) sugar

2 ½ Tbsp (37 mL) sweet rice flour

½ tsp (2 mL) cinnamon

⅛ tsp (0.5 mL) salt

dash of nutmeg

½ cup (125 mL) raisins, soaked (optional)

1 Tender Pie Crust (top and bottom; see page 114)

Egg Wash

1 large egg, room temperature (see page 6), beaten

1 Tbsp (15 mL) milk

Preheat oven to 450°F (230°C). Add lemon juice to apples and toss to prevent browning. Pour water into a pot large enough to hold apples and heat on medium.

Mix next 5 ingredients. Add to water and boil, constantly stirring, for about 2 minutes. Add apples and raisins and return to a boil. Simmer over low for 5 to 6 minutes until apples are tender. Pour filling into prepared pie crust.

Beat egg in a small bowl and add milk. Brush edges of pie crust with egg wash and top with second pie crust. Using a knife, make small slits in top layer of pie. Brush top with egg wash. Bake in preheated oven for 15 minutes. Reduce heat to 350°F (175°C). Bake for another 30 to 35 minutes until filling has thickened.

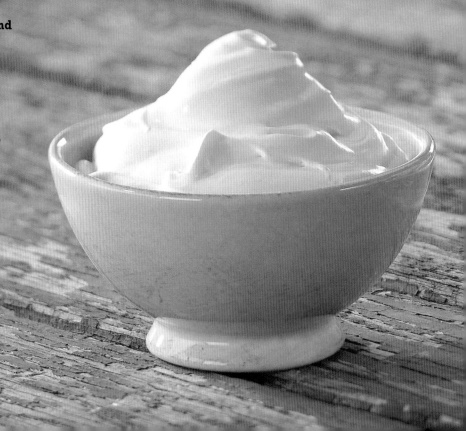

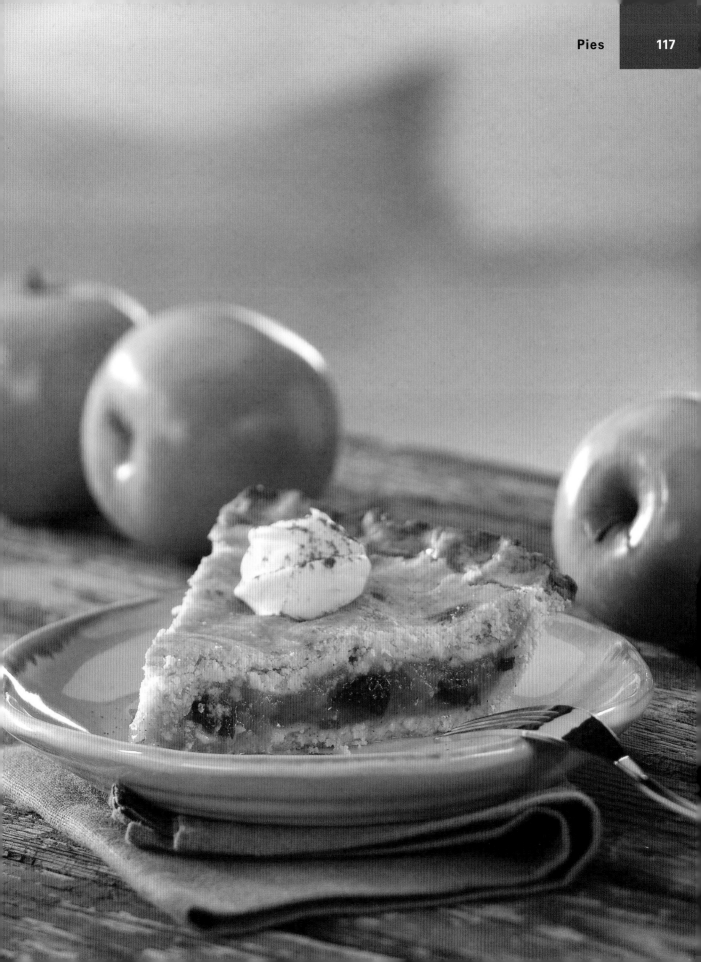

Blueberry Pie

Cuts into 8 wedges

Just the beautiful look of all these blueberries makes me want to break out the spoon and start eating. I always use wild berries for better texture and flavour.

4 to 5 cups (1 to 1.25 L) blueberries (wild preferred)

½ cup (125 mL) sugar

2 ½ Tbsp (37 mL) sweet rice flour

1 Tbsp (15 mL) lemon juice

¼ tsp (1 mL) cinnamon

1 Tender Pie Crust (top and bottom; see page 114)

1 Tbsp (15 mL) butter

Egg Wash

1 large egg, room temperature (see page 6)

1 Tbsp (15 mL) milk

sugar, for sprinkling

Preheat oven to 450°F (230°C). Mix together first 5 ingredients.

Pour filling into first prepared pie crust. Dot butter on top of filling.

Beat egg in small bowl and add milk. Brush edges of pie crust with egg wash and top with a second pie crust. Using a knife, make small slits in top layer of pie.

Brush top with egg wash and sprinkle with sugar. Bake in preheated oven for 15 minutes. Reduce heat to 350°F (175°C). Bake for another 30 minutes until filling has thickened.

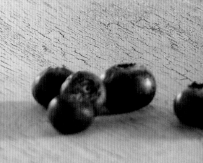

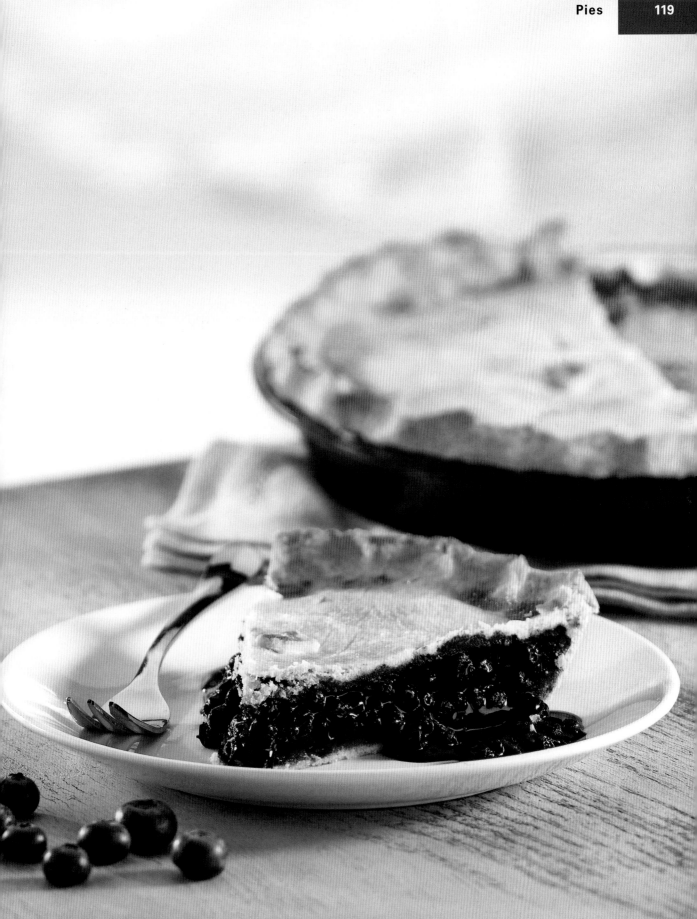

Saskatoon Pie

Cuts into 8 wedges

One of the most-loved Canadian specialties. I go out every year hunting for the plumpest saskatoon berries just to be able to make this pie. I prefer the smaller wild to the orchard type, but both will work well.

4 cups (1 L) saskatoon berries

¾ cup (175 mL) sugar

2 ½ Tbsp (37 mL) sweet rice flour

1 Tender Pie Crust (top and bottom; see page 114)

1 Tbsp (15 mL) butter

Egg Wash

1 large egg, room temperature (see page 6)

1 Tbsp (15 mL) milk

sugar, for sprinkling

Preheat oven to 450°F (230°C). Mix together first 3 ingredients.

Pour filling into first prepared pie crust. Dot butter on top of filling.

Beat egg in a small bowl and add milk. Brush edges of pie crust with egg wash and top with a second pie crust. Using a knife, make small slits in top layer of pie.

Brush top with egg wash and sprinkle with sugar. Bake in preheated oven for 15 minutes. Reduce heat to 350°F (175°C). Bake for another 30 to 35 minutes until filling has thickened.

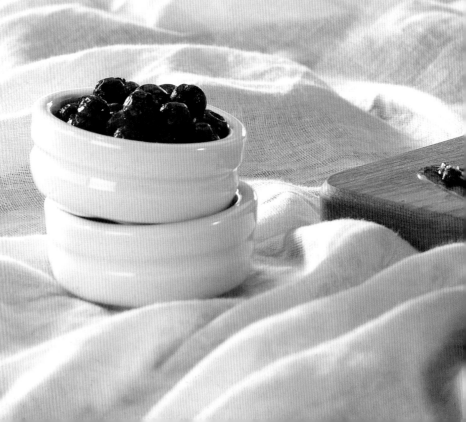

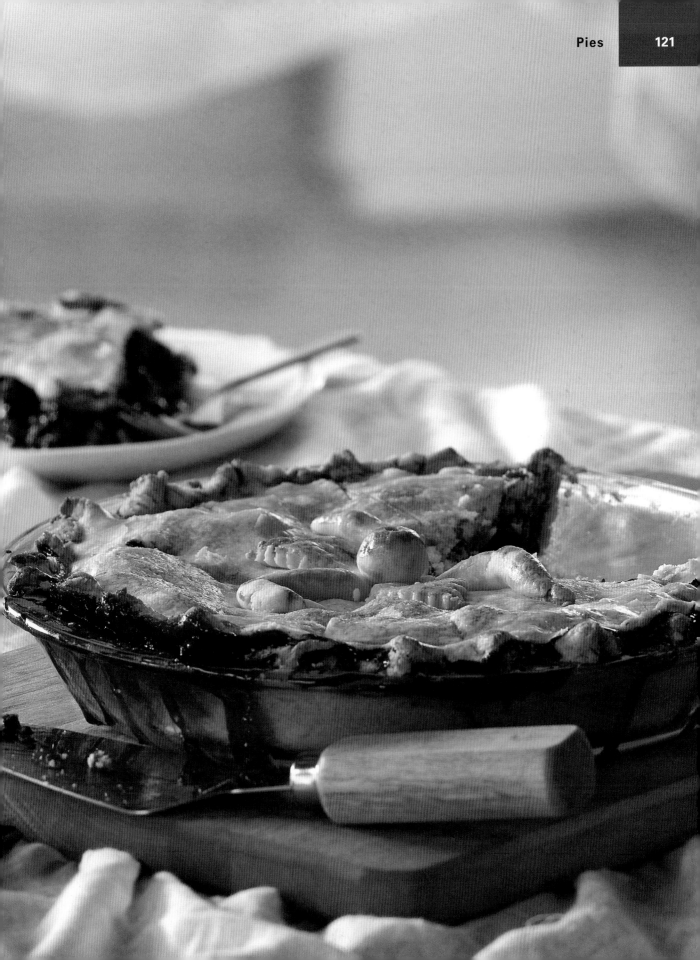

Lemon Meringue Pie

Cuts into 8 wedges

An classic old-time pie that is a favourite of children. It looks pretty and is fun to make.

2 cups (500 mL) water

1 ¼ cups (300 mL) sugar

6 Tbsp (90 mL) cornstarch

½ tsp (2 mL) salt

4 egg yolks, room
temperature (see page 6)

½ cup (125 mL) lemon
juice

3 Tbsp (45 mL) butter

1 Tbsp (15 mL) lemon zest

1 Tender Pie Crust,
prebaked (bottom only; see
page 114)

Meringue Topping

4 egg whites, room
temperature (see page 6)

6 Tbsp (90 mL) sugar

Mix first 4 ingredients in a 8 cup (2 L) pot. Heat over medium for 3 minutes, stirring constantly to prevent burning. Remove from heat.

Beat egg yolks in a bowl. Add ½ cup (125 mL) hot mixture a little at a time, stirring. Add egg yolk mixture to remaining hot mixture in pot. Bring to a gentle boil for 3 minutes, stirring constantly. Remove from heat.

Stir in next 3 ingredients. Let cool.

Pour filling into prebaked pie crust. Place in refrigerator and cool until set.

Preheat oven to 350°F (175°C). Beat egg whites in medium bowl until soft peaks form. Add sugar, 1 Tbsp (15 mL) at a time, beating constantly until stiff peaks form. Spread meringue on set lemon pie, covering pie to edges. Bake in preheated oven for about 10 minutes until meringue reaches desired browning.

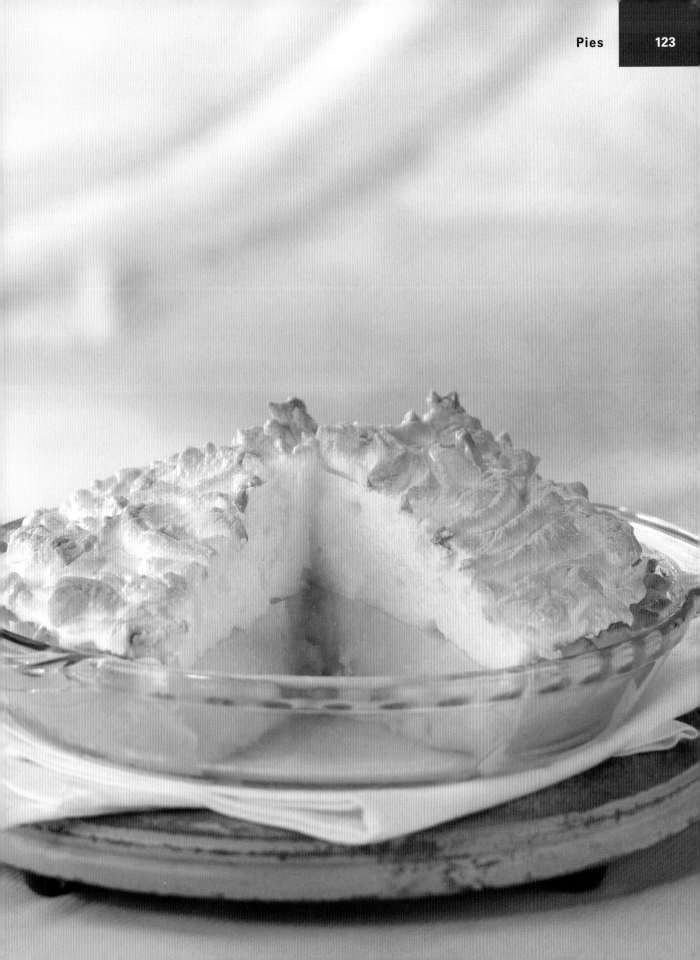

Chocolate Chip Cookies

Makes 5 ¹/₂ dozen

A decadent and soft chocolate chip cookie that will become an easy-to-make family favourite. Loaded with chocolate chips.

³⁄₄ cup (175 mL) white rice flour

¹⁄₂ cup (125 mL) pea starch

¹⁄₂ cup (125 mL) yellow corn flour

¹⁄₄ cup (60 mL) sorghum flour

¹⁄₄ cup (60 mL) tapioca starch

1 tsp (5 mL) baking soda

³⁄₄ tsp (4 mL) xanthan gum

¹⁄₂ tsp (2 mL) salt

1 cup (250 mL) butter, softened

³⁄₄ cup (175 mL) light brown sugar

³⁄₄ cup (175 mL) sugar

1 tsp (5 mL) vanilla

2 large eggs, room temperature (see page 6)

2 cups (500 mL) semi-sweet chocolate chips

1 cup (250 mL) chopped walnuts or pecans (optional)

Preheat oven to 375°F (190°C). Mix first 8 ingredients in a large bowl.

Beat next 4 ingredients in an extra-large bowl until creamy. Add eggs 1 at a time, beating well after each addition. Add flour mixture until well combined.

Add chocolate chips and nuts. Drop 2 tsp (10 mL) scoops onto ungreased cookie sheets. Bake in preheated oven for 8 to 10 minutes until lightly browned. Remove from oven and let cool slightly. Transfer cookies from cookie sheets to wire racks to cool completely.

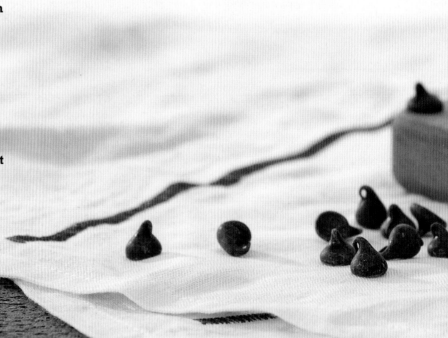

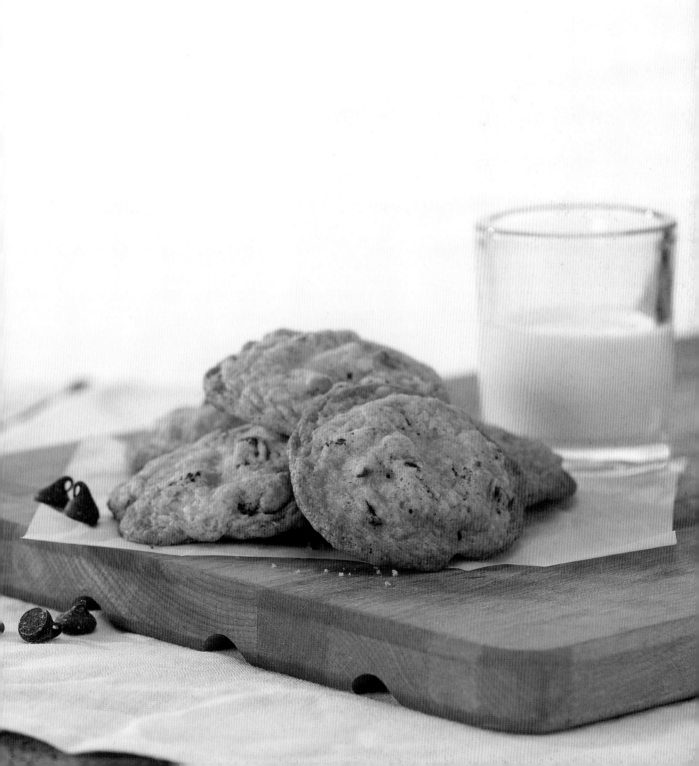

Sorghum, a relative of corn, is gaining popularity among gluten-free bakers. It is also wildly used by gluten-free beer breweries.

Fudgy Chocolate Chip Cookies

Makes 4 dozen

A chewy, fudgy variation of an old-time classic chocolate chip cookie. These cookies stay soft for a long time. Brown sugar and milk chocolate chips lend a decadent burst of flavour.

¾ cup (175 mL) white rice flour

½ cup (125 mL) yellow corn flour

¼ cup (60 mL) pea starch

¼ cup (60 mL) sorghum flour

¼ cup (60 mL) tapioca starch

1 tsp (5 mL) baking soda

½ tsp (2 mL) xanthan gum

⅛ tsp (0.5 mL) salt

2 cups (500 mL) brown sugar

⅔ cup (150 mL) butter, softened

1 tsp (5 mL) vanilla

2 Tbsp (30 mL) hot water

2 large eggs, room temperature (see page 6)

1 cup (250 mL) milk chocolate chips

Preheat oven to 350°F (175°C). Mix first 8 ingredients in a large bowl.

Beat next 3 ingredients in an extra-large bowl until creamy. Add hot water. Add eggs 1 at a time, beating well after each addition. Add flour mixture until well combined.

Add chocolate chips. Chill dough for 30 to 60 minutes in refrigerator. Drop 2 tsp (10 mL) scoops onto ungreased cookie sheets. Bake cookies in preheated oven for 8 to 10 minutes until lightly browned. Remove from oven and let cool slightly. Transfer cookies from cookie sheets to wire racks to cool completely.

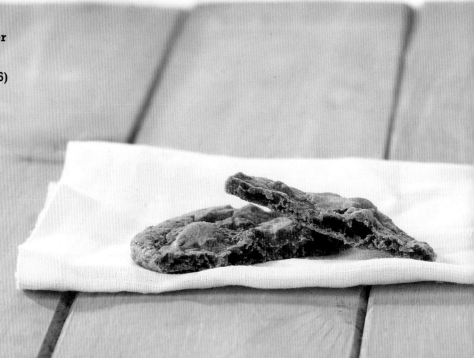

Great food prepared in the company of great music makes for a wonderful combination. Sometimes an artist strikes a chord inside and you find yourself listening to their music over and over again. While working on this book, I found myself listening to a new emerging artist from Canada, Alex Vissia. Her masterful songwriting, haunting melodies and powerful voice make a perfect blend, just like a good recipe. Check her out at alexvissia.com when you have time. I am particularly fond of "Wild Fig Tree" and "Goodnight Moonlight" from her album A Lot Less Gold.

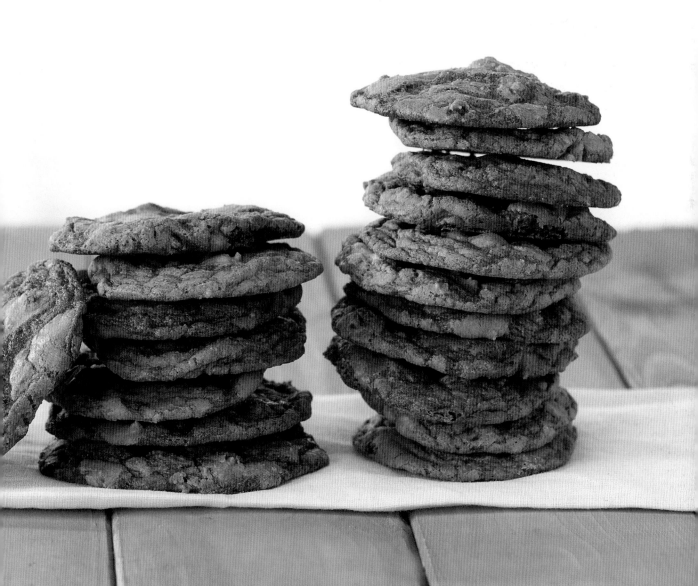

Gingersnaps

Makes 7 dozen

The all-time seasonal winner in the cookie category. A crisp, thin and flavourful spiciness combines with the deep undertone of molasses.

1 cup (250 mL) white rice flour

¾ cup (175 mL) pea starch

¼ cup (60 mL) sorghum flour

¼ cup (60 mL) yellow corn flour

2 tsp (10 mL) ginger

1 tsp (5 mL) baking soda

1 tsp (5 mL) cinnamon

1 tsp (5 mL) xanthan gum

½ tsp (2 mL) cloves

¼ tsp (1 mL) salt

1 cup (250 mL) butter, softened

1 cup (250 mL) berry sugar, plus ¼ cup (60 mL) for rolling

1 tsp (5 mL) vanilla

1 large egg, room temperature (see page 6)

¼ cup (60 mL) molasses (see Tip)

Preheat oven to 350°F (175°C). Mix first 10 ingredients in a large bowl.

Beat butter, 1 cup (250 mL) sugar and vanilla in an extra-large bowl until creamy. Add egg and molasses and beat well. Add flour mixture and beat until well combined. Chill dough for 2 hours in refrigerator. Dough will be stiff. Form 1 inch (2.5 cm) balls, roll in remaining sugar and place onto ungreased cookie sheets. If you bake one sheet at a time, chill dough in between batches. Bake in preheated oven for 12 to 15 minutes until cookies are slightly darker at edges and show tiny cracks on surface. Remove from oven and let cool slightly. Transfer cookies from cookie sheets to wire racks to cool completely.

Tip

You can use fancy or blackstrap molasses, according to your preference. I personally like to use blackstrap.

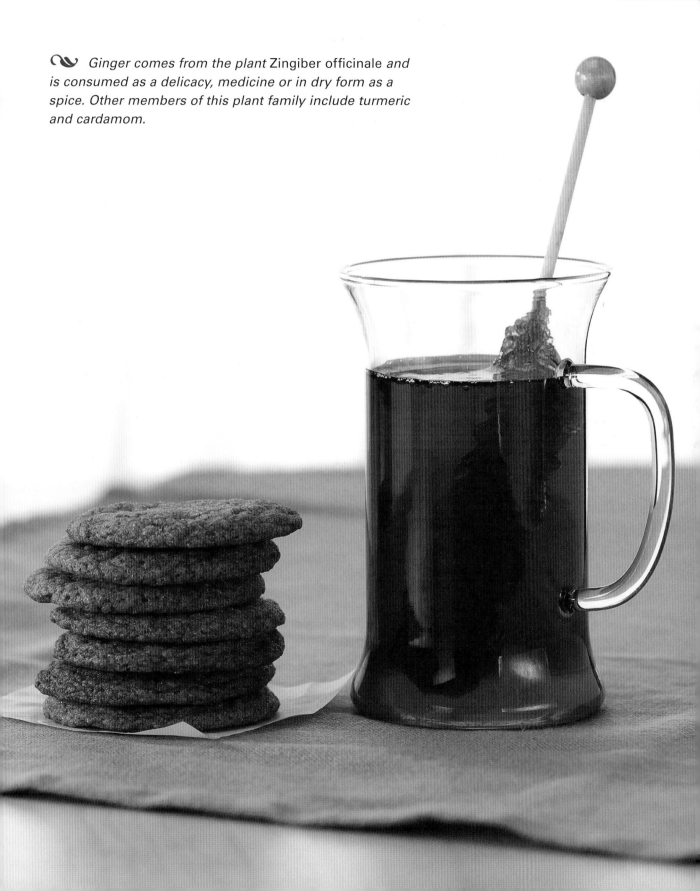

Ginger comes from the plant Zingiber officinale *and is consumed as a delicacy, medicine or in dry form as a spice. Other members of this plant family include turmeric and cardamom.*

Chocolate-dipped Corn Cookies

Makes 2 dozen

A European shortbread cookie with the unique combination of yellow corn flour, orange flavouring and a complementary chocolate covering. These easy-to-make cookies store well for a long time (if you can keep them away from hungry mouths).

2 cups (500 mL) yellow corn flour

1 tsp (5 mL) baking powder

½ tsp (2 mL) xanthan gum

¾ cup (175 mL) sugar

½ cup (125 mL) butter, softened

½ cup (125 mL) shortening

2 large eggs, room temperature (see page 6)

½ tsp (2 mL) orange flavouring

½ tsp (2 mL) vanilla

1 cup (250 mL) chocolate wafers, melted

Preheat oven to 375°F (190°C). Mix first 3 ingredients in a large bowl.

Beat next 3 ingredients in an extra-large bowl until creamy. Add eggs 1 at a time, beating well after each addition. Add orange flavouring and vanilla. Add flour mixture and beat until well combined. Using a teaspoon, drop onto ungreased cookie sheets and flatten with a fork. Bake in preheated oven for 8 to 10 minutes. Remove from oven and let cool slightly. Transfer cookies from cookie sheets to wire racks to cool completely.

Dip ⅓ to ½ of each cookie into melted chocolate or drizzle chocolate over top. Place on wire racks to set.

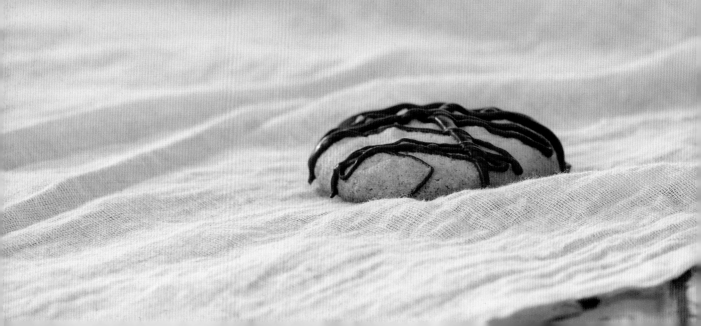

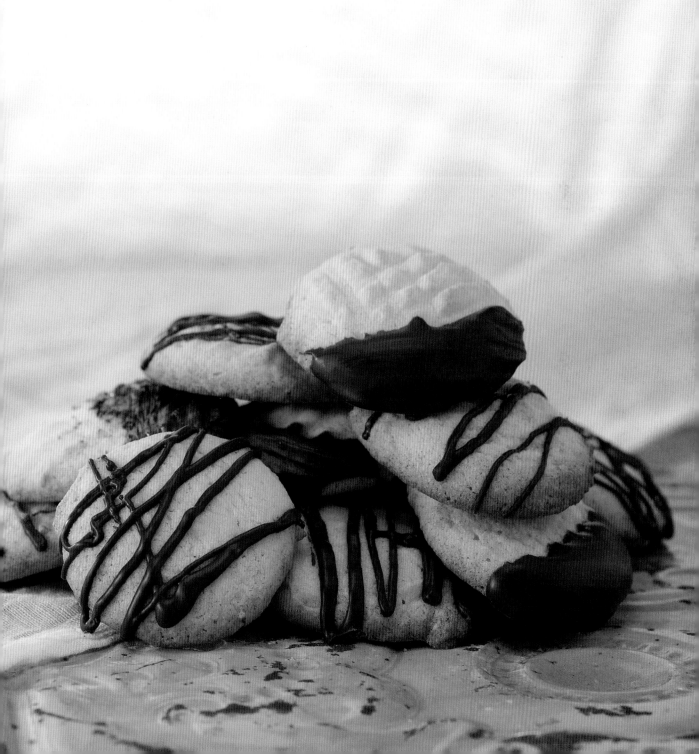 *To melt chocolate wafers, heat them slowly in the microwave in 20 second installments until they're completely melted. Don't heat the chocolate for too long at a time, or you might end up with a burned mess.*

Shortbread Cookies

Makes 4 dozen

The perfect company for a cup of tea. This cookie offers the traditional richness of timeless decadence.

1 cup (250 mL) cornstarch

1 cup (250 mL) white rice flour

2 Tbsp + ¾ tsp (34 mL) potato starch

2 Tbsp + ¾ tsp (34 mL) tapioca starch

½ tsp (2 mL) xanthan gum

1 cup (250 mL) butter-flavoured shortening

½ cup (125 mL) icing sugar

1 tsp (5 mL) vanilla

Preheat oven to 325°F (160°C). Mix next 5 ingredients in a large bowl.

Beat shortening in an extra-large bowl until creamy. Add icing sugar and beat well. Add vanilla. Add flour mixture and beat until well combined. Press or roll dough out on table lightly floured with rice flour to ¾ to 1 inch (2 to 2.5 cm) thickness. Cut dough into desired shapes and prick with a fork. Bake in preheated oven for 15 to 20 minutes until just golden. Remove from oven and let cool slightly. Transfer cookies from cookie sheets to wire racks to cool completely.

The texture of shortbread is "short" or crumbly as a result of the high fat to starch (or flour) ratio.

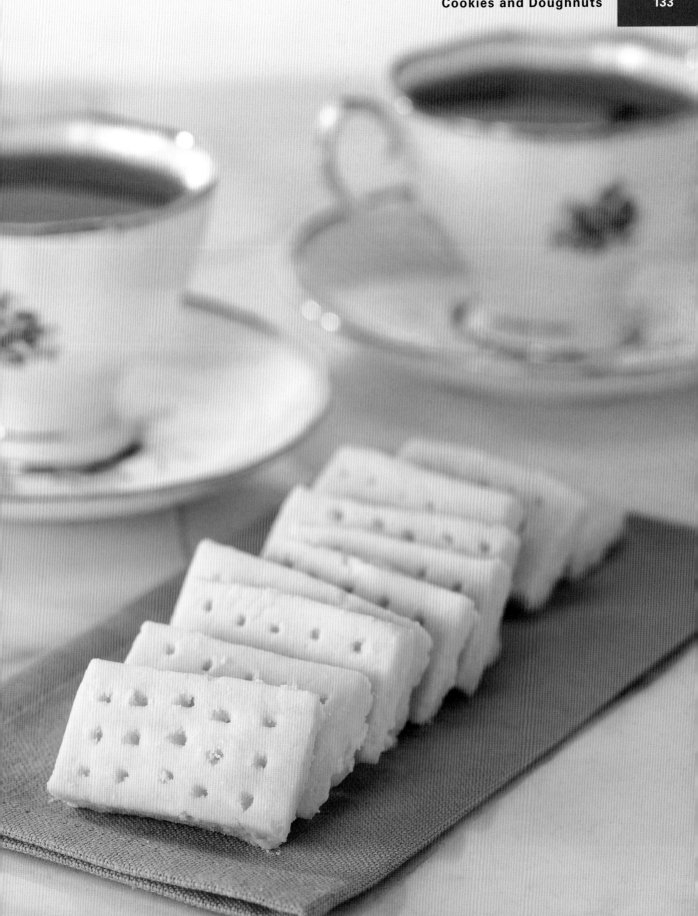

Bird's Nest Cookies

Makes 3 dozen

With their colourful display of toasted coconut edges and jam-filled centres, these shortbread-style cookies will not last long enough to store!

1 ⅓ cup (325 mL) flaked coconut

1 cup (250 mL) white rice flour

½ cup (125 mL) cornstarch

¼ cup (60 mL) potato starch

¼ cup (60 mL) tapioca starch

½ tsp (2 mL) xanthan gum

1 cup (250 mL) butter

½ cup (125 mL) sugar

1 large egg, room temperature (see page 6)

½ tsp (2 mL) vanilla

raspberry jam or red glazed cherries

Preheat oven to 300°F (150°C). Spread coconut on ungreased baking sheet. Toast in preheated oven for 15 to 18 minutes until golden brown. Remove from oven. Increase oven temperature to 350°F (175°C).

Mix next 5 ingredients in a large bowl.

Beat butter in an extra-large bowl until creamy. Add sugar and beat well. Add egg, vanilla and flour mixture and beat well. Form dough into 1 ¼ inch (3 cm) balls. Roll in toasted coconut. Flatten onto cookie sheet.

Make imprint with thumb in middle of each cookie. Add raspberry jam or glazed cherry into indent. Bake in preheated oven for 12 to 15 minutes until golden. Remove from oven and place on a wire rack to cool.

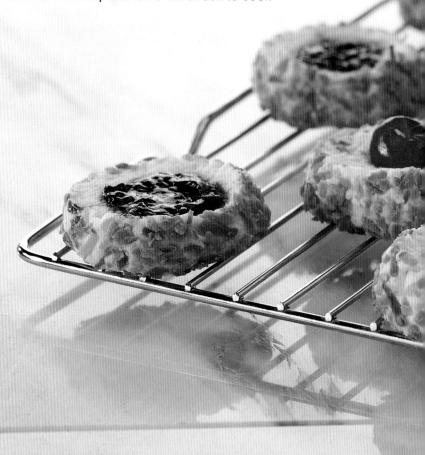

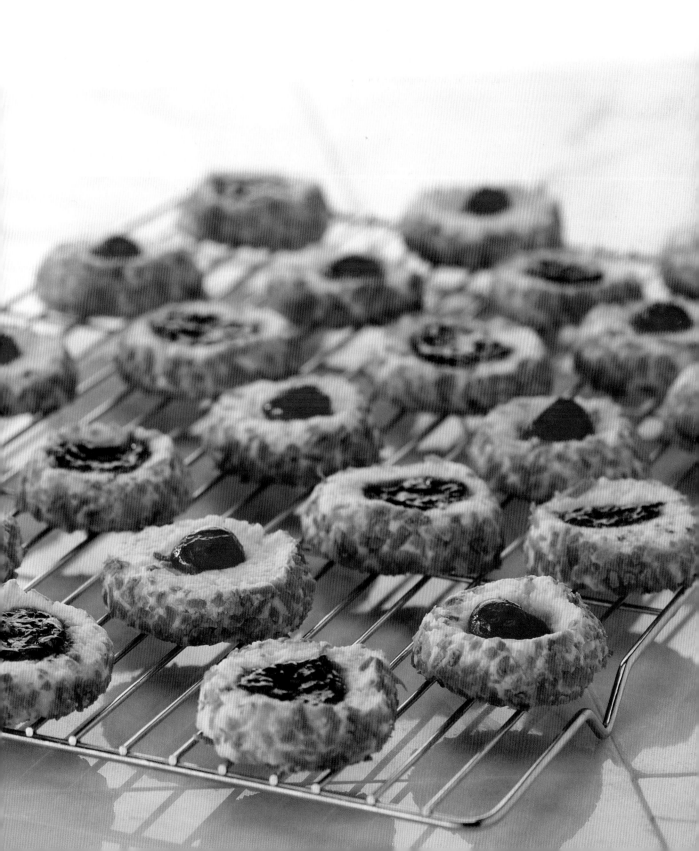

Sugar Cookies

Makes 3 dozen

Colourful decorations on these traditional sugar cookies add an eye-pleasing display to your treat platter. These crisp, tender cookies easily cut into your favourite shapes. These are light sugar cookies, but they can be decorated if they're handled lightly.

4 cups (1 L) potato starch

¼ cup (60 mL) tapioca starch

2 tsp (10 mL) baking powder

½ tsp (2 mL) salt

½ tsp (2 mL) xanthan gum

1 cup (250 mL) butter-flavoured shortening

1 ½ cup (375 mL) sugar

4 egg yolks, room temperature

1 tsp (5 mL) orange flavouring

1 tsp (5 mL) vanilla

coloured sprinkles

Preheat oven to 350°F (175°C). Mix first 5 ingredients in a large bowl.

Beat shortening in an extra large bowl until creamy. Add sugar and beat well. Add next 3 ingredients and starch mixture and beat well. Turn out dough onto surface lightly floured with sweet rice flour. Roll to ½ inch (12 mm) thickness. With cookie cutters, cut into desired shapes and place on ungreased cookie sheets.

Decorate with sprinkles. Bake in preheated oven for 9 to 12 minutes until just golden. Remove from oven and let cool slightly. Transfer cookies from cookie sheets to wire racks to cool completely.

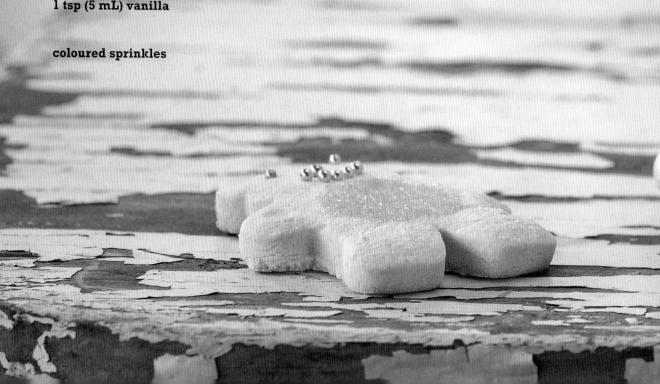

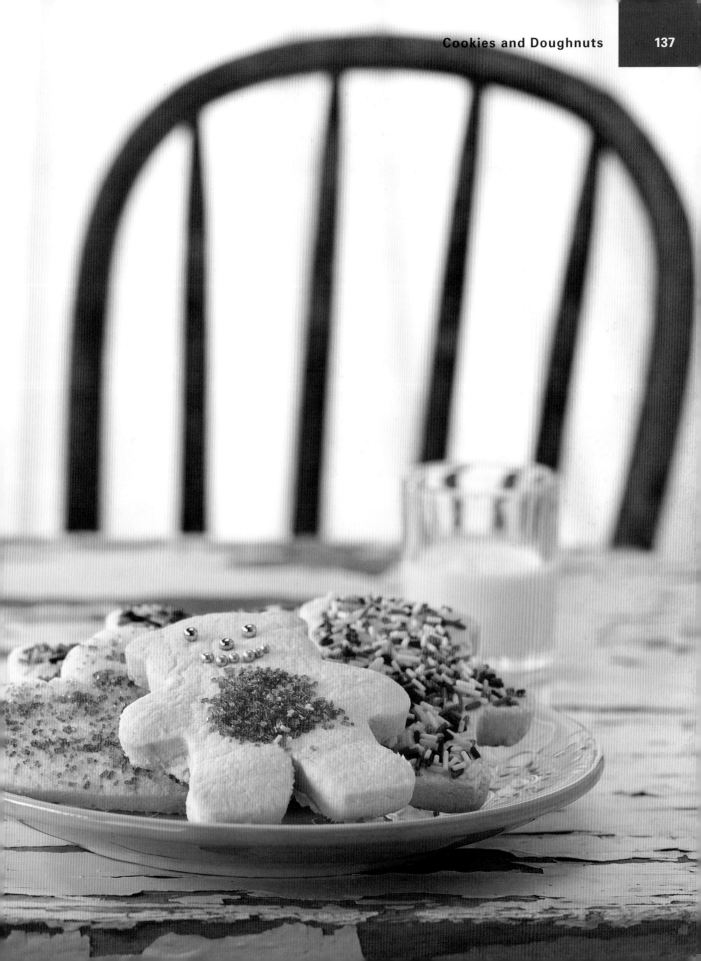

Cranberry Almond Cookies

Makes 4 ¹/₂ dozen

Sliced almonds and flavourful cranberries make for a sure winner that doesn't just tantalize your taste buds, but also your eyes.

³⁄₄ **cup (175 mL) white rice flour**

¹⁄₂ **cup (125 mL) pea starch**

¹⁄₂ **cup (60 mL) yellow corn flour**

¹⁄₄ **cup (60 mL) sorghum flour**

¹⁄₄ **cup (60 mL) tapioca starch**

1 Tbsp (15 mL) pea fibre 80

1 tsp (5 mL) baking soda

³⁄₄ **tsp (4 mL) xanthan gum**

¹⁄₂ **tsp (2 mL) salt**

1 cup (250 mL) butter, softened

³⁄₄ **cup (175 mL) light brown sugar**

³⁄₄ **cup (175 mL) sugar**

1 tsp (5 mL) lemon flavouring

1 tsp (5 mL) vanilla

2 large eggs, room temperature (see page 6)

2 cups (500 mL) dried sweetened cranberries

1 cup (250 mL) thinly sliced almonds

Preheat oven to 350°F (175°C). Mix first 9 ingredients in a large bowl.

Beat next 5 ingredients in an extra-large bowl until creamy. Add eggs 1 at a time, beating well after each addition. Add flour mixture and beat until well combined.

Add cranberries and almonds. Drop 2 tsp (10 mL) scoops onto ungreased cookie sheets. Bake in preheated oven for 8 to 10 minutes until lightly browned. Remove from oven and let cool slightly. Transfer cookies from cookie sheets to wire racks to cool completely.

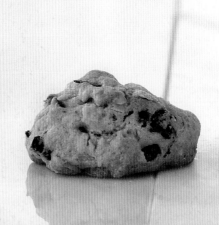

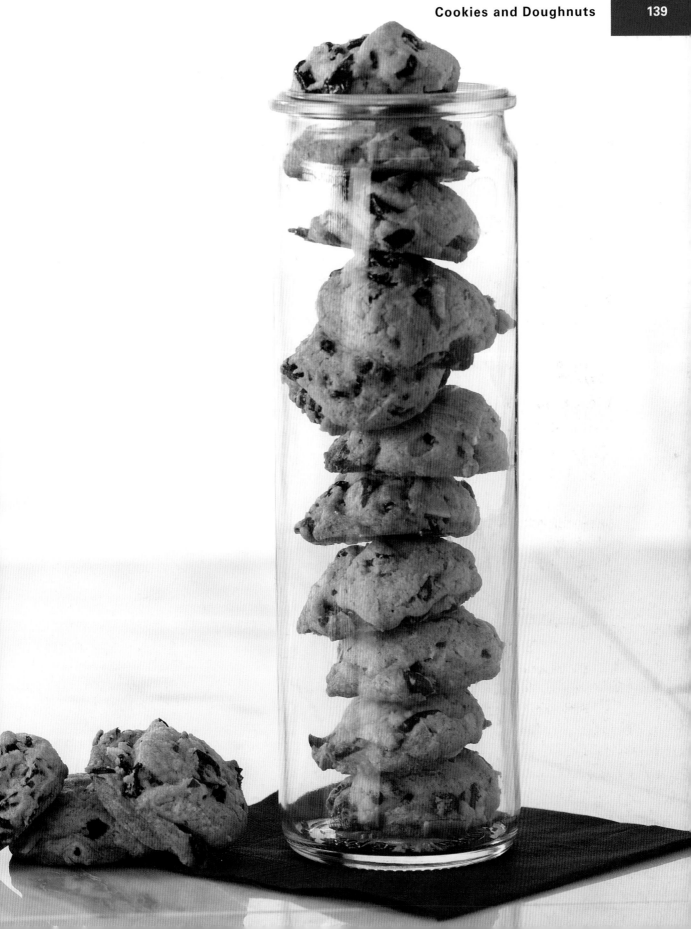

Drop Doughnuts

Makes about 3 dozen

A fast and easy cake-style doughnut that makes a great afternoon snack. These are best eaten shortly after frying.

lard, for frying

1 cup (250 mL) white rice flour

½ cup (125 mL) pea starch

¼ cup (60 mL) tapioca starch

¼ cup (60 mL) yellow corn flour

2 Tbsp (30 mL) sugar

2 tsp (10 mL) baking powder

2 tsp (10 mL) xanthan gum

½ tsp (2 mL) nutmeg

½ tsp (2 mL) salt

4 egg yolks (large), room temperature

1 large egg, room temperature (see page 6)

1 ¾ cup (425 mL) milk (or almond milk)

¼ cup (60 mL) oil

2 tsp (10 mL) vanilla

1 cup (250 mL) berry sugar, for coating

Heat lard to 350°F (175°C) in a deep fryer.

Mix first 9 ingredients in an extra-large bowl.

Blend next 5 ingredients in a separate bowl. Add egg mixture to flour mixture and mix until batter is smooth. Using a teaspoon, drop batter into preheated fat. Flip doughnuts when they rise to the surface. Fry for about 2 ½ minutes. I fry mine until they're golden brown; adjust the frying time to your liking. Remove doughnuts from fryer and drop onto paper towel to absorb excess fat.

While still warm, roll or coat doughnuts in berry sugar. Place on wire rack to cool (unless you want to eat them right then and there!).

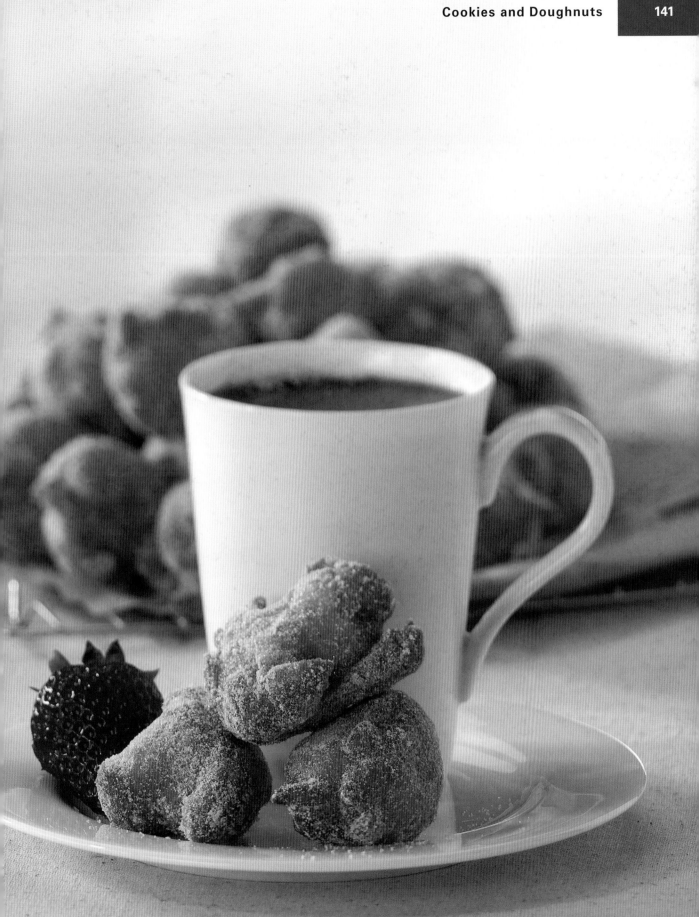

Apple Fritters

Makes 15 to 24

These are one of my all-time favourite doughnuts, with their funny shape, soft texture and perfect balance of sweetness and spice. Make sure to use fresh spices.

lard, for frying

1 cup (250 mL) icing sugar, for coating

1 to 2 Tbsp (15 to 30 mL) warm water

1 cup (250 mL) white rice flour

½ cup (125 mL) sweet rice flour

¼ cup (60 mL) tapioca starch

¼ cup (60 mL) yellow corn flour

2 Tbsp (30 mL) sugar

1 Tbsp (15 mL) xanthan gum

2 tsp (10 mL) baking powder

2 tsp (10 mL) instant yeast

½ tsp (2 mL) cinnamon

½ tsp (2 mL) nutmeg

½ tsp (2 mL) salt

1 cup (250 mL) coarsely grated apple

4 egg yolks (large), room temperature

1 large egg, room temperature (see page 6)

1 cup (250 mL) warm milk

¼ cup (60 mL) oil

2 tsp (10 mL) vanilla

Heat lard to 350°F (175°C) in a deep fryer.

Mix icing sugar and water in a small bowl. Set aside.

Mix next 12 ingredients in an extra-large bowl.

Blend last 5 ingredients in a separate bowl. Add egg mixture to flour mixture. Mix until batter is smooth. Let stand for 20 minutes. Using a tablespoon, drop batter into preheated fat. Flip fritters when they rise to the surface. Fry for about 2 ½ to 3 minutes. I fry mine until they're golden brown; adjust the frying time to your liking. Remove fritters from deep fryer and drop onto paper towel to absorb excess fat. While still warm, coat in icing sugar mixture. Place on wire racks to cool. (In our house, somehow there are very few left for cooling.)

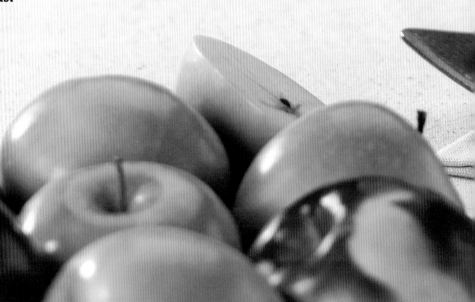

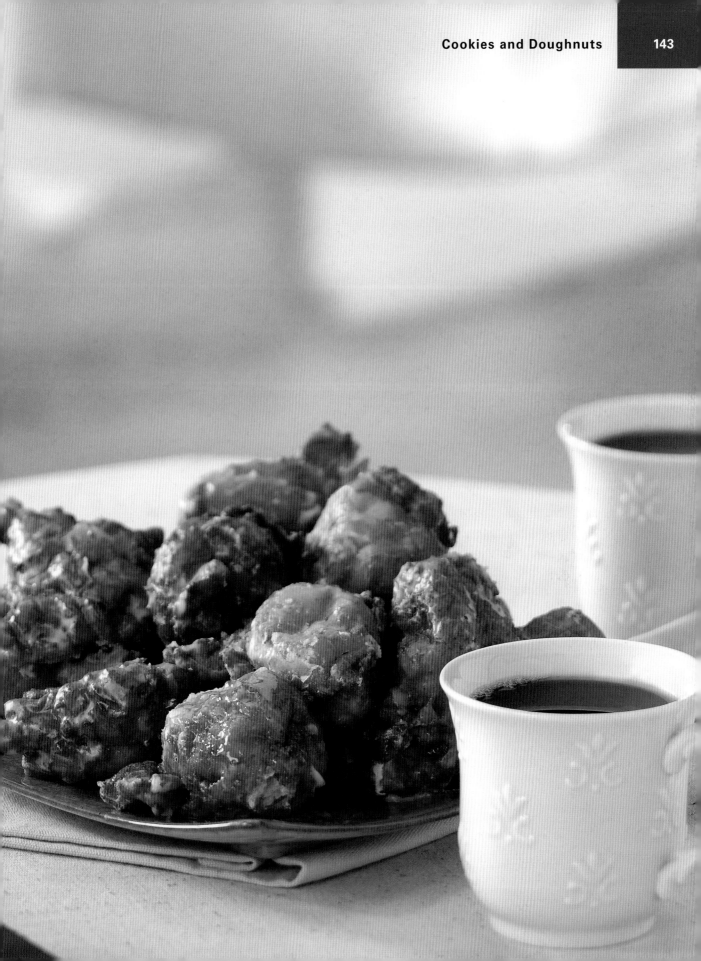

Yeast Doughnuts

Makes about 12

An airy and light doughnut that is worth the wait of the yeast rising. These doughnuts expand nicely in the deep fryer. If you're adventurous, try filling them with jam.

lard, for frying

1 cup (250 mL) berry sugar

1 tsp (5 mL) cinnamon

1 cup (250 mL) white rice flour

1/2 cup (125 mL) pea starch

1/4 cup (60 mL) tapioca starch

1/4 cup (60 mL) yellow corn flour

2 Tbsp (30 mL) sugar

4 tsp (20 mL) xanthan gum

1 Tbsp (15 mL) instant yeast

2 tsp (10 mL) baking powder

1 tsp (5 mL) dough improver (see page 19)

1/2 tsp (2 mL) salt

1/2 tsp (2 mL) nutmeg

1/4 cup (60 mL) oil

4 egg yolks (large), room temperature

1 large egg, room temperature (see page 6)

2 tsp (10 mL) vanilla

1 1/4 cup (300 mL) very warm milk

Heat lard to 350°C (175°C) in a deep fryer.

Mix berry sugar and cinnamon in a small bowl. Set aside.

Mix next 11 ingredients in an extra-large bowl.

Blend last 5 ingredients in a separate bowl. Add egg mixture to flour mixture. Mix until dough is smooth. Turn out onto surface lightly floured with white rice flour. Roll out to about 1/2 inch (12 mm) thickness. Cut out doughnuts to desired size with a doughnut cutter (I cut mine to about 3 inches [7.5 cm]). Place doughnuts on a baking sheet. Place in a warm place and cover with a damp towel. Let rise for about 20 minutes. Drop doughnuts into preheated fat. Flip doughnuts when they rise to the surface. Fry for about 2 1/2 to 3 minutes. I fry mine until they're golden brown; adjust the frying time to your liking. Remove doughnuts from fryer and drop onto paper towels to absorb excess fat. While still warm, coat in berry sugar mixture. Place on wire racks to cool.

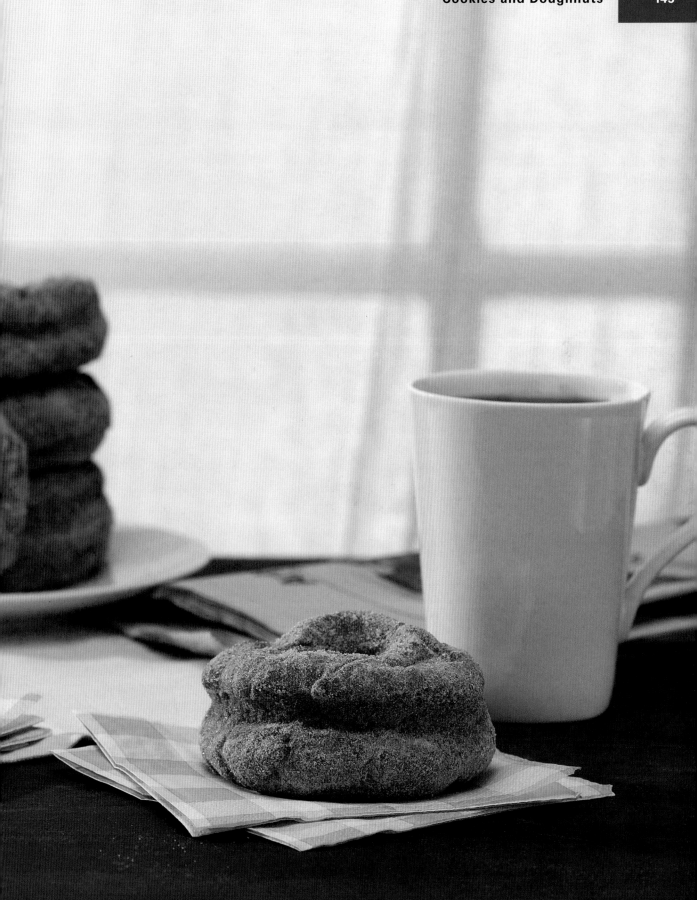

Pancakes

Makes about 2 dozen

Light and fluffy, with a perfect colour, texture and taste. Pass the maple syrup and fresh raspberries!

1 cup (250 mL) white rice flour

$\frac{1}{2}$ cup (125 mL) pea starch

$\frac{1}{4}$ cup (60 mL) tapioca starch

$\frac{1}{4}$ cup (60 mL) yellow corn flour

2 Tbsp (30 mL) sugar

1 $\frac{1}{2}$ tsp (7 mL) baking powder

1 tsp (5 mL) xanthan gum

$\frac{1}{2}$ tsp (2 mL) salt

2 cups (500 mL) milk

2 large eggs, room temperature (see page 6)

$\frac{1}{4}$ cup (60 mL) oil

2 tsp (10 mL) vanilla

butter (optional)

Mix first 8 ingredients in an extra-large bowl.

Blend next 4 ingredients in a separate bowl. Add egg mixture to flour mixture. Mix until batter is smooth. Let stand for 10 minutes. Preheat griddle to medium. I add a bit of butter to the griddle. Drop batter onto griddle, using about 2 Tbsp (30 mL) for each pancake. Cook until bubbles form on top, then flip pancake. Cook for 2 $\frac{1}{2}$ to 3 minutes until golden.

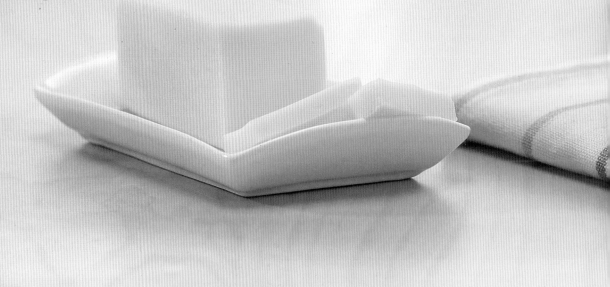

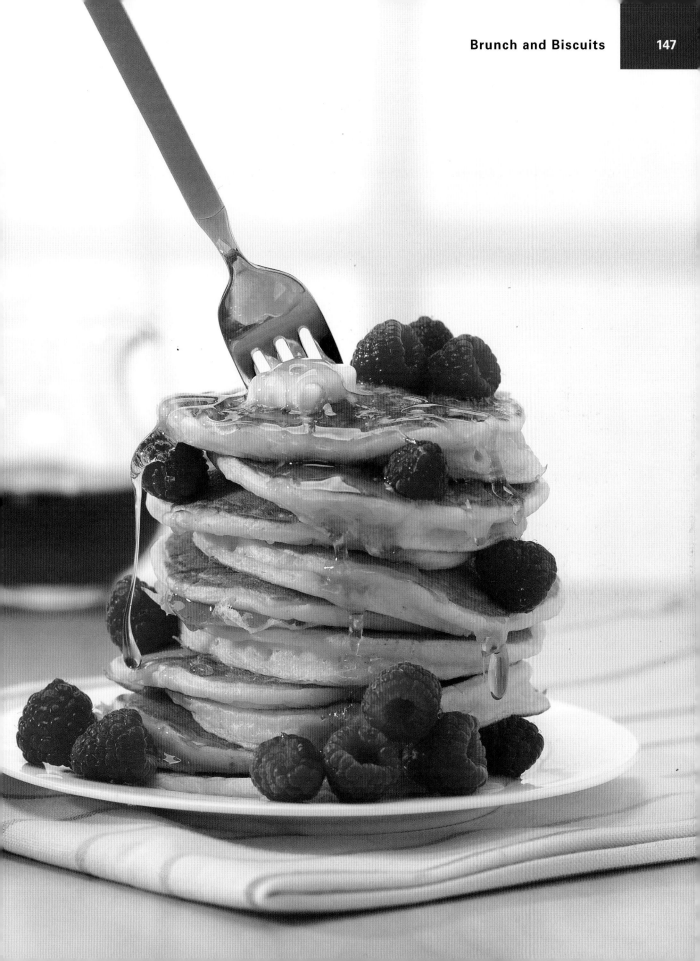

Waffles

Makes 12 to 15

Why limit waffles to breakfast time? We make these beautiful, tender waffles any time of the day that we desire. Serve with your favourite toppings, such as syrup or blueberries.

2 Tbsp (30 mL) egg whites, room temperature

1 cup (250 mL) white rice flour

½ cup (125 mL) pea starch

¼ cup (60 mL) tapioca starch

¼ cup (60 mL) yellow corn flour

3 Tbsp (45 mL) sugar

1 ½ tsp (7 mL) baking powder

1 tsp (5 mL) xanthan gum

½ tsp (2 mL) salt

2 ½ cups (625 mL) milk

¼ cup (60 mL) oil

2 large eggs, room temperature (see page 6)

2 tsp (10 mL) vanilla

butter (optional)

Beat egg whites in a small bowl until stiff.

Mix next 8 ingredients in an extra-large bowl.

Blend next 4 ingredients in a separate bowl. Add egg mixture to flour mixture. Mix until batter is smooth. Fold in egg whites. Let stand for 10 minutes. Follow your waffle maker instructions and drop batter by the suggested volume on preheated waffle griddle. I use butter in my griddle first. Adjust waffle baking time to achieve desired crispness.

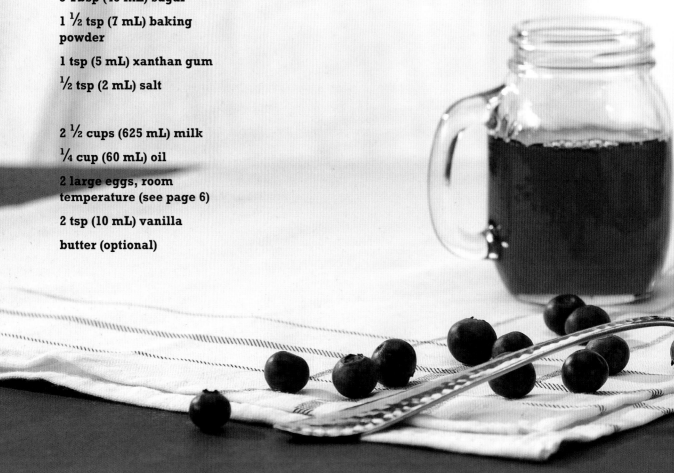

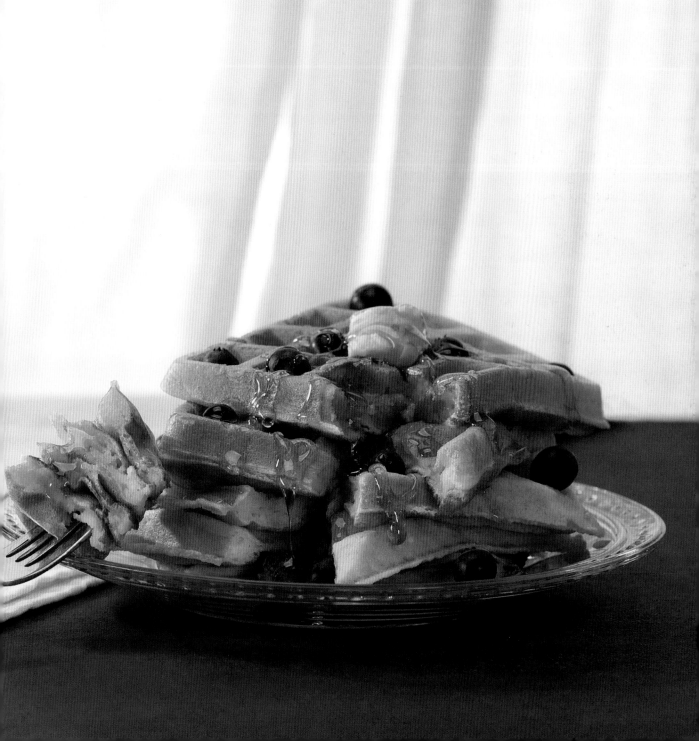

Belgian waffle irons that have a turnable base are popular among bakers because they make an even-textured, fluffy waffle. I find that this waffle recipe turns out well in just about any waffle maker.

European Thin Pancakes

Makes 12 to 15

These ever-so-tender crepe-like pancakes are reminiscent of Swedish or German fare. Fill them with your favourite jam, fruit or cream, or like many of us try them with Nutella or lemon juice and sugar. I also use these thin pancakes with savoury fillings to make a wrap.

½ cup (125 mL) white rice flour

¼ cup (60 mL) pea starch

2 Tbsp (30 mL) sugar

2 Tbsp (30 mL) tapioca starch

2 Tbsp (30 mL) yellow corn flour

1 tsp (5 mL) xanthan gum

½ tsp (2 mL) salt

2 cups (500 mL) milk (or almond milk)

3 large eggs, room temperature (see page 6)

2 Tbsp (30 mL) oil

2 tsp (10 mL) vanilla

butter (optional)

Mix first 7 ingredients in an extra-large bowl.

Blend next 4 ingredients in a separate bowl. Add egg mixture to flour mixture. Mix until batter is smooth. Let stand for 10 minutes. Preheat griddle to medium. I add a bit of butter to the griddle. Drop batter onto griddle, using about 2 Tbsp (30 mL) for each pancake. Spread out batter into a flat circle. Cook until bubbles form on top, then flip pancake. Cook for about 2 to 3 minutes until golden. These pancakes are thin and can be rolled up with your favourite filling.

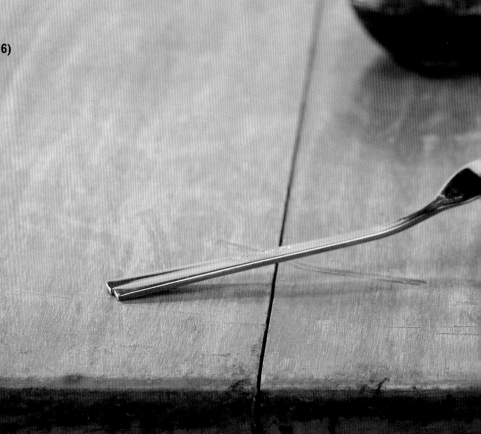

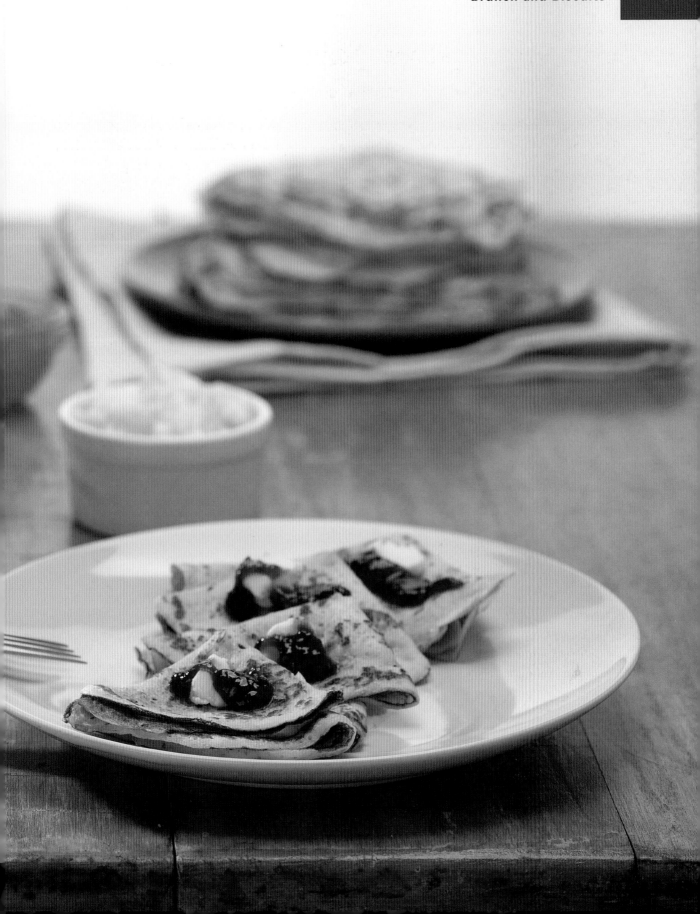

Tea Biscuits

Makes 8 to 12

Tea time, coffee time, breakfast time, supper. Any time can be tea biscuit time!

1 cup (250 mL) white rice flour

½ cup (125 mL) tapioca starch

⅓ cup (75 mL) pea starch

1 ½ Tbsp (25 mL) baking powder

1 tsp (5 mL) salt

1 tsp (5 mL) xanthan gum

½ cup (125 mL) shortening

¾ to 1 cup (175 to 250 mL) milk

Egg Wash
1 large egg, room temperature (see page 6)

1 Tbsp (15 mL) milk

Preheat oven to 400°F (200°C). Mix first 6 ingredients in a large bowl.

Cut shortening into dry mixture until a fine crumb consistency. Add milk and work in with a fork until a soft dough is formed. Turn out dough onto surface lightly dusted with white rice flour. Roll out to ½ to ¾ inch (12 mm to 2 cm) thickness. Cut out circles with lightly floured biscuit or cookie cutter. Place on a greased baking sheet.

Mix together egg and milk. Brush biscuits with egg wash. Bake in preheated oven for 12 to 15 minutes until golden brown. Serve while still warm with Devonshire cream and jam.

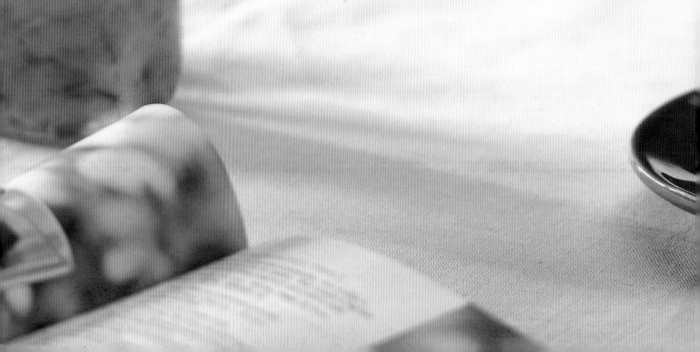

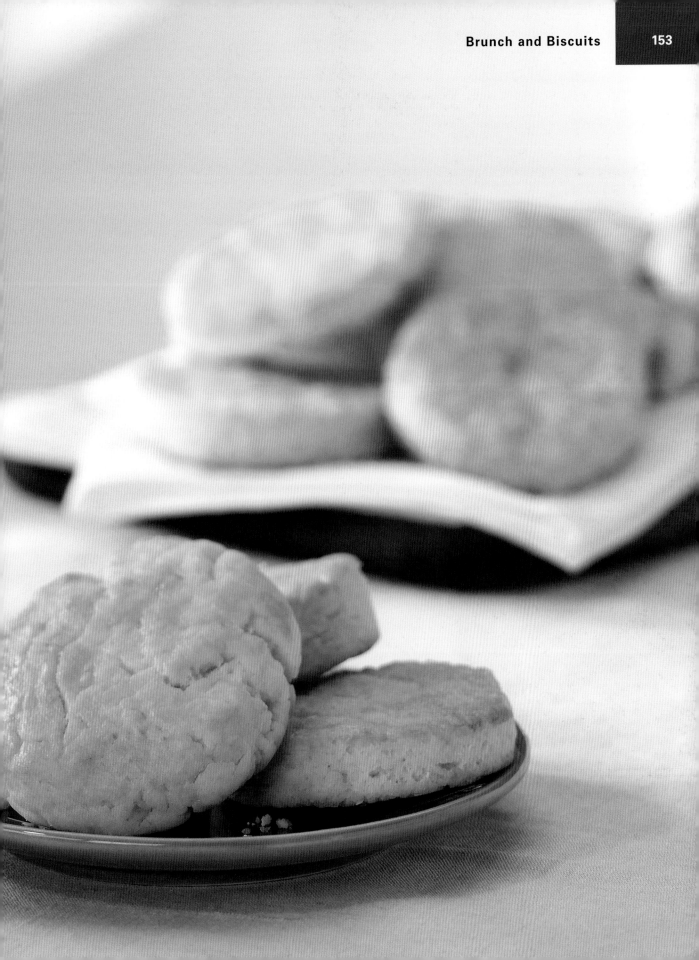

English Muffins

Makes 8 to 12

A perfect companion to Eggs Benedict, or you can just use them as a bun anytime.

¼ cup (60 mL) warm water

1 Tbsp (15 mL) active dry yeast

2 tsp (10 mL) sugar

1 cup (250 mL) potato starch

1 cup (250 mL) tapioca starch

1 cup (250 mL) white rice flour

¼ cup (60 mL) whey powder

2 Tbsp (30 mL) pea fibre 80

4 tsp (20 mL) sugar

1 Tbsp (15 mL) xanthan gum

1 tsp (5 mL) dough improver (see page 19)

1 tsp (5 mL) salt

1 ½ cups (375 mL) water

½ cup (125 mL) egg whites, room temperature

¼ cup (60 mL) oil

fine cornmeal for dusting

Place first 3 ingredients in a small bowl. Let stand for 10 minutes until foamy.

Thoroughly mix next 9 ingredients in an extra-large bowl.

Blend next 3 ingredients in a separate bowl. Add egg white mixture and yeast mixture to flour mixture. Mix until a smooth batter is formed.

Sprinkle cornmeal on bottom of greased 3 inch (7.5 cm) round bun pans. Pour batter into pans and smooth with a wet spatula. Place in a warm place and cover with a damp towel. Let rise until about doubled in size. Place pans in a 400°F (200°C) oven on middle rack. Bake for 15 minutes. Flip buns upside down in pan. Bake for another 15 minutes until firm and slightly golden. Remove pan from oven. Place buns upside down on a wire rack to cool.

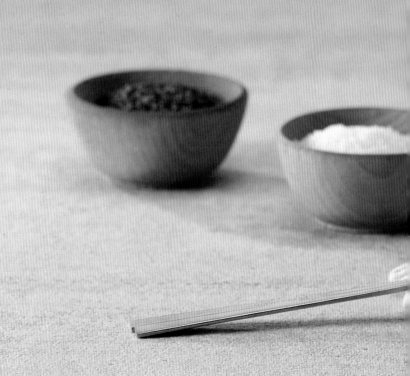

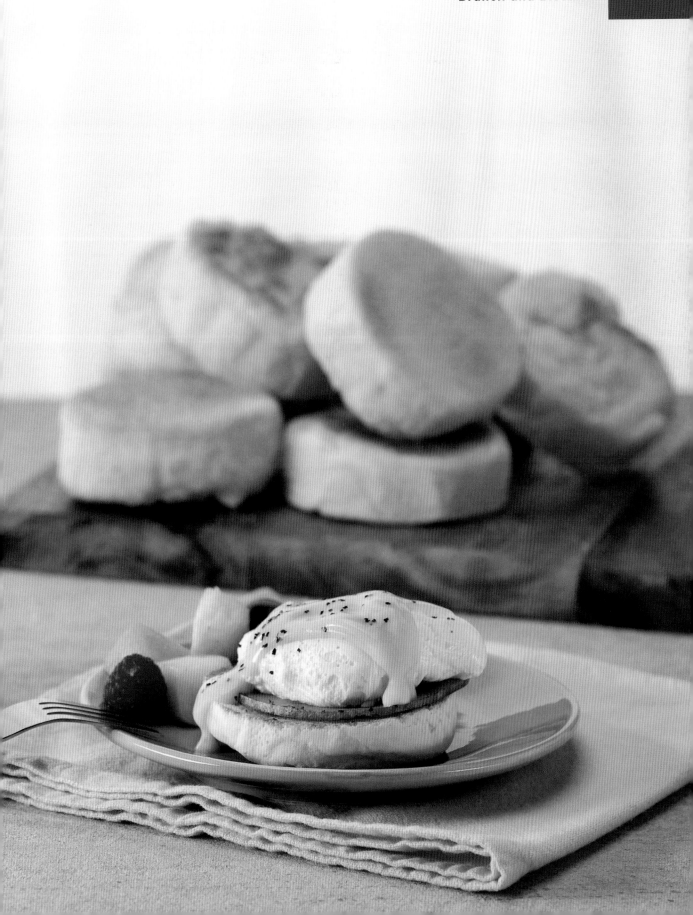

Raisin English Muffins

Makes 8 to 12

Raisins, cinnamon and sorghum blend well in this morning delight.

¼ cup (60 mL) warm water

1 Tbsp (15 mL) yeast

2 tsp (10 mL) sugar

1 cup (250 mL) tapioca starch

1 cup (250 mL) white rice flour

¾ cup (175 mL) raisins

½ cup (125 mL) potato starch

½ cup (125 mL) sorghum flour

¼ cup (60 mL) whey powder

2 Tbsp (30 mL) pea fibre 80

4 tsp (20 mL) sugar

1 Tbsp (15 mL) xanthan gum

1 tsp (5 mL) baking powder

1 tsp (5 mL) cinnamon

1 tsp (5 mL) dough improver (see page 19)

1 tsp (5 mL) salt

1 ½ cups (375 mL) water

½ cup (125 mL) egg whites, room temperature

¼ cup (60 mL) oil

fine cornmeal

Preheat oven to 400°F (200°C). Place first 3 ingredients in a small bowl. Let stand for 10 minutes until foamy.

Thoroughly mix next 13 ingredients in an extra-large bowl.

Blend next 3 ingredients in a separate bowl. Add egg white mixture and yeast mixture to flour mixture. Mix until a smooth batter is formed.

Sprinkle cornmeal on bottom of greased 3 inch (7.5 cm) round bun pans. Pour batter into greased pans and smooth with a wet spatula. Place in a warm place and cover with a damp towel. Let rise until doubled in size. Place pans in preheated oven on middle rack. Bake for 15 minutes. Flip buns upside down in pan. Bake for another 15 minutes until firm and slightly golden. Remove pan from oven. Place buns upside down on a wire rack to cool.

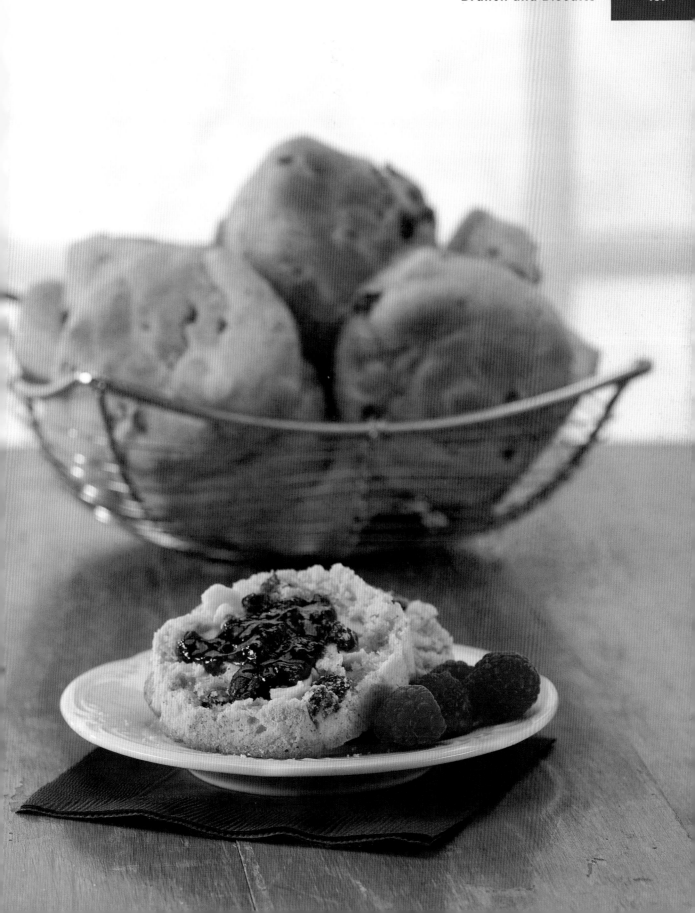

Index

Acknowledgements

The book you are holding and reading, like any good thing in life, is the product of many great people coming together and embarking on a journey to create something special.

The vibrant energies that I've encountered in putting this book together are many and are frankly quite amazing. The many thousands of customers that I had the pleasure of meeting over many years as founder and former owner of internationally renowned gluten-free manufacturer Kinnikinnick Foods Inc. are the driving force for this book. To the many business partners and colleagues in the gluten-free food-manufacturing world, I applaud you for providing more and more great-tasting gluten-free products.

Foremost, I thank my loved ones for being there from the beginning to the completion of this book. Your endless taste-testing, love and support means everything. You know who you are.

To my many friends who tasted hundreds of recipes over the years: you kept me motivated and encouraged me to write the book—and you all learned to not double dip!

Thank you to all the absolutely brilliant people at Company's Coming whose creativity, vision and enthusiasm extend beyond any book. I had the honour of meeting and working with so many of you, too many to list all of you. Know that I thank all of you for being part of this project. To name a few, I would like to thank Linda Dobos for her help in preparing the recipes for the photo sessions, and for noticing that maybe that 4 Tbsp of baking powder should possibly read 4 tsp. I know you, the reader, will appreciate this.

I also thank Ashley Billey for her countless hours of helping with the preparation of the recipes and her absolutely amazing food-styling skills. She can make a banana peel look like a crème brûlée.

Thank you to my main photographer Sandy Weatherall for her incredible vision, her desire for perfection, her creative focus and unsurpassed photography skills. She makes me want to bite into the book.

I also thank Kelsey Attard and Nancy Foulds, the editors who put up with my Germanized English and put my creative vision into a printable format.

A big thank you to the very visionary owners of Company's Coming for making this book a reality.

Last but not least, I'd like to thank the creative director of Catalyst Theatre, without whom none of this might have happened.